MORE
HYPNOTIC SCRIPTS THAT WORK
The Breakthrough Book - Volume 2
by
John Cerbone, CHt, BCH, CI

Another Hypnosis Script Encyclopedia for Professional Hypnotists

→ Featuring 70+ Original Hypnotic Suggestion Breakthrough Scripts
→ 10+ Pages of Topic Specific "Extras"
→ 88 Session Optimizing Suggestions (SOS) for a Variety of Subjects

Your Insider Secret to Session Success!

This is the sequel to the book that Ormond McGill, the Dean of American Hypnotists called: "A Wonderful, Wonderful Work! Something every modern Hypnotist must have (for use) in their practice!"

MORE HYPNOTIC SCRIPTS THAT WORK
The Breakthrough Book - Volume 2
By John Cerbone, CHt, BCH, CI

Text Copyright © 2011 by John Cerbone, Cerbone Hypnosis Institute
Editing and Cover Design by Paula Duncan Nongard

ISBN #

First Printing July 2011
Printed in the United States of America
Expert Author Publishing
http://www.expertauthorpublishing.com/

John Cerbone – Cerbone Hypnosis Institute
CerboneHypnosisInstitute.com   Trance-Master.com
HypnotistPro.com   FastestHypnotistAlive.com

TABLE OF CONTENTS

WEIGHT LOSS AND HEALTH 96

SMOKING CESSATION 135

PERSONAL DEVELOPMENT 143

SPORTS PERFORMANCE ENHANCEMENT 183

RELATIONSHIPS 195

BEER & ALCOHOL 209

Session Optimizing Statements (SOS) 215

Foreword

Thank you for purchasing this updated edition of my book: ***More Hypnotic Scripts That Work, The Breakthrough Book*** – Volume 2.

This text represents years of my work in the field of clinical hypnosis. As a trained and well-seasoned hypnotic professional, I have come to use deepening techniques, truisms and confusion method strategies within these suggestion scripts to further deepen the hypnotic state while the client (patient) is hypnotized, to increase impact and long-term effectiveness.

These scripts and techniques are written in the style and language of this profession, including *run-on sentences, redundancy, and specific yet sometimes grammatically incorrect language patterns,* which is the way most true hypnosis professionals verbally deliver suggestions for greatest impact. In other words, they do not read like a short story; they read like a hypnosis script should.

All of the original suggestions, techniques and methods contained herein have been used with actual clients and were proven effective and beneficial, quite often achieving remarkable results in one or just a few sessions. Subsequently, you may very likely find your clients achieving breakthroughs quite rapidly.

Important Notes: As with any professional tool, it is assumed and understood that you will be pre-reading each of the scripts before using them so that you are familiar with the content and language patterns, and that you will make any necessary and appropriate adjustments based upon the specific needs of the individual client.

You may want to utilize an entire script, or just certain sections for addressing a specific issue.

In this edition, in addition to the **88 Session Optimizing Statements (SOS's)** at the end, I've also included several *Extras* sections, which is a grouping of various suggestions I've written targeted to specific client weak spots on specific subjects, to insure greater lasting, high-impact success. You could piece several of them together to formulate and fill in a script, or select individual phrases or statements to drop into your own script to drive home a powerful point.

In closing, I wish to sincerely thank my clients, my family, loved ones, friends and colleagues for their tireless support and inspiration, which has helped to make this work possible. I wish to also thank all of those individuals with whom I have trained over the years and all of those practitioners who have gone before me, as well as those who represent the future of these noble professions.

And as a purchaser of this work, I want to sincerely and personally thank you for your interest and support. I truly wish you and those whose lives you help to improve through your service and dedication, limitless creative inspiration and unstoppable success in each and every area of your lives.

Sincerely,

John Cerbone
Board Certified Hypnotist
Certified Clinical Hypnosis Instructor
Master Hypnotist

CerboneHypnosisInstitute.com
Trance-Master.com
HypnotistPro.com
FastestHypnotistAlive.com

CAUTION:

This book is solely and strictly intended for use only by professionals in the field of hypnosis, including but not necessarily limited to professionally trained: Hypnotherapists, Clinical Hypnotists, Psychologists, Psychotherapists, Psychoanalysts, Psychiatrists and other skilled Mental Health Professionals, who have been properly trained and certified in the use of professional/clinical hypnosis.

This information is being shared so that people will be helped, lives will be improved and so other professionals as listed above can experience enhanced benefit and improvement from their work into the world.

Every state has different rules and regulations concerning the practice of hypnosis. In certain states, some client conditions may fall under the heading of "medical" or "mental health" treatment, and you must be a qualified and certified Clinical Hypnosis professional and have a written note of authorization from the client's attending physician, psychiatrist, psychologist, etc., to perform certain complementary hypnosis sessions, with no exceptions.

It is up to the individual hypnotist to perform appropriately within the scope of their training and state governance.

Stress, Fears and Situational Control

Stress Free, Past Releases and Forgiven

As you relax, your automatic mind now is retooled, re-tuned, reset, re-calibrated, to respond differently and better, in a brand new and better chapter of your life, taking better care of you, feeling more supportive, and more trusting in each and every moment.

As slow and steady regular deep and soothing breath begins to take place, as the new habit pattern for release, you begin to truly trust in your life.

The way it is now creating itself around you, through each and every thought, now more supportive, you now more forgiving, healed, and released.

A new and safer sense of peace and serenity now surround and embrace you, and as if magically, you relax , and automatically recognize that your breathing now guides your way to a new and better more peaceful and supported existence.

Gone now and forever, in this brand new and certainly true chapter of your life, are the days you once felt stressed out, as your automatic mind, is now unbeatably and even heroically, working in your favor, automatically, in ways both known and unknown to you, to relax you, restore you, empower you.

Your life just seems to flow, every word, every thought, every habit, every action, every self-supporting reaction, generates a greater sense of relief, release, and serenity both in and out of you.

You're breathing now more steady, your heart rate now more peaceful and serene, as you now and forever create a life and existence that supports you, both day and night.

Now more safe and sure of yourself, trusting in this you now know this to be true, almost as if guided from on high somewhere, almost as if, a light from somewhere now comes down around you, the golden-white soothing healing blanket of restoration unconditional love joy, and ecstatic feelings, creating a more comfortable you.

This soothing, healing, light, regenerating and restoring you, releasing the past, becoming one with you, melting into every molecule, and fiber that is you, balancing and restoring you, both physically and emotionally, mentally and spiritually.

A new harmony and alignment now felt and known within you, truly you now know, any and all things past that once blocked were hindered, you now released, releasing, forgiven and gracefully and directly moving on, now knowing this to be true, more and more, more and more, on each and every breath and heartbeat.

As you relax even deeper now, memorizing the sense of peace, relaxation, rest, more easily able to deep breathe, as slow and steady breath, strengthens and guides you, generating serenity and inner and outer peace, to release, and regenerate serenity for you.

While you are awake, while you are asleep, while you are dreaming, happy pleasant dreams, happy pleasant thoughts, overwhelm the limitations of the past, and you and now as peaceful and calm, even creatively creating this, certain and sure you are now free.

Almost as if from deep, deep inside of you, it's like someone has reset a switch, the dial, the thermostat, or reset a computer of some kind, opened a valve of some sort, draining away what no longer needs to be there, and restore it if only putting back in its place, all that needs to be.

What others think of you is only their business, and none of your business, to each their own, and you forever now move on.

Each and every night before bedtime, a new regimen for a better life begins. All of the day's issues and struggles, all of the day's worries and challenges, relaxed away from, put upon a shelf.

Free now forever your mind is and becomes, never stressing over these things, the day put up on a shelf an hour into each and every night before bedtime, as you simply go to bed, put your head on the pillow and just go to sleep, like thousands of times before in your past.

Your mind is now working any and all of this out in your favor, in the most self-supporting of ways, you are now your own best friend, any and all of this working out in ways both known and unknown to you, and so it is and remains forever on each and every slow and steady breath and heartbeat.

Any challenge, any and all things from the past, your mind now releasing, and letting go of, just as you have moved on from the ways of your childhood, so too you have moved on most assuredly from any and all of that, truly released, forgiven, and healed, it happens automatically on its own, feeling and getting to experiment in order to improve this sense of serenity, peace, and life support.

Any and all past challenges which no longer serve you, truly now no longer serve and are released, now forgiven truly, and you moving on.

By letting go of the past, you forgive it, release it, and sweep it aside, making room, for the masterpiece of a life in an existence, you now more truly and absolutely generate create yourself, taking anything and everything in stride, truly you now, at peace.

Like a mighty river cascading down the side of the mountain in the spring, with a boulder in the center of that river, any and all challenge, stress and adversity simply flows around you and polishes you in the process, you now a mighty master of your life, and determined to forever remain so.

You know, any and all of this becoming easier and better each and every time you do it, deeper and better rest, deeper and better peace, almost as if each and every time you repeat this enjoyable relaxation stayed on your own, you are doing perhaps sixteen to eighteen years worth of healing in the deepest and most truest sense.

Your life simply better and better, slow and steady deep breathing guides your way.

Self-Confidence – Relief and Empowerment

As you relax, float, drift and dream, your whole body melts and relaxes, as you enter in ways very best, both known and unknown to you, truly, and amazingly forever, a brand new and better chapter of your life.

In this brand new and better place, you are relaxed, in your own skin, you have relaxed, to any and all formerly now done barriers, into a greater and wider plane and space, a greater method of existence, a greater perception of your improved life.

A more fulfilling sense of self now begins to blossom.

All things once disruptive or imbalanced, now released, now relieved, now let go of, into the past, like a sunrise in the morning, warming your skin, warming you inside and out.

A brand new and better chapter has now risen up and shined down upon you into your life, generating peace and light, restoring a greater sense of harmony, trust, self-assured and truly knowing this, more now than ever before, not because I say so, but because it is in fact true, for in this new chapter of your life, you breakthrough and thrive, or have simply relax and succeed, and you now know this to be undeniably true.

Your new correct and forever response to high stress is deep breaths slowly taken and released, generating unstoppable deep and profound, truest serene relaxation.

As you once let go of the things of your youth, in favor of your adulthood, so too now and forever, your adaptive, reactive, and now working in your favor mind, every thought, each and every feeling, each and every action, each and every reaction, restores harmony, generates light in and out of you.

Vanquishing any and all stress or even discomfort, regret, forever renewed, forever freed of sabotage, restoring tranquility, life force, health, and a more beautiful life, as you now have released imbalance, and in its place, restoring harmony and balance in the very best and most unstoppable of ways, so automatic, so effective, instantly and aggressively responsive, that your only option is feeling better, good, mighty, rising up, facing down challenges effectively.

Free at long last, into the very best chapter and moments of your life, for the past now is gone, forgiven, released, healing, whole, and self-perfecting all that you do, are, and remain becoming, with each and every beat of your heart, with each and every word that I say.

With every pulse of your eyelids, any and all of this, now you rejuvenated, retained, re-tuned, reset, reinvented, reinvigorated, even at times clever and heroic, just loving yourself creatively, more and better, releasing, each and every day, in the masterpiece way, to break you through, and to free you.

Right now is the time, and right now is your point of power, as your energy is tuned up, activated, turned on, having grown up just a little bit more, almost as if having done effectively, the work of fifteen to eighteen years worth of healing, right now in this moment.

And each and every time you do these enjoyable relaxation techniques on your own, you step powerfully and undeniably forward, to seize each moment, to live your life, to free yourself, to cut yourself a break, and to love yourself, unconditionally, in ways meaningful, the way an ideal parent would love a wonderful and innocent child, so nurturing, so loving, more joy and laughing, ever expanding.

For the greater the challenge once was, the more reconditioned and empowered, even inspired, moreover divinely guided you become.

Polishing up your life, you now create and invent ways to take very much better care of yourself.

Your now restored and self-correcting mind, can do what it chooses, in this new chapter of your life, this powerful unstoppable mind of yours, thinks about how supportive your life has actually been, by virtue of the fact that you are here and meant to be here, and visualizes life's lessons for yourself and your loved ones, and the most supportive and gentle of ways, beneficial outcomes, now more and more your own.

You now knows this to be true.

Seeing the past is now done and released, healing, and forgiven, each and every second, each and every blink of your eyes, each and every beat of your heart, each and every breath, each and every time you do this technique on your own, a greater reminder, both steadying and calming, as greater and greater feelings of serenity and peace are now within you, you make this your own.

Creative and clever now your mind, continually building forward in this, even a shortfall or a stumble, something you can now more easily laugh at, forgive, let go of, and release, feeling relief, serenity and peace now your own, so easily, adaptively, and cleverly created.

Ahhhh, released and relaxed.

Trusting in your life, now more confident in beneficial outcomes, trusting in you, more confidence now your own.

For the greater the challenge, the mightier and more cleverly adaptive, effective and breakthrough you become.

Relaxing with yourself, alone or with others, calm and tranquil, you relax, and open your heart and mind, like a fountain of light, to loving yourself as well as other people, your face, heart and mind, now and forever shine in radiant, glowing, growing, life force.

More and more flow, you come and go, most especially in social moments, a time to share your light and shine

Inner wisdom now blossoms, the past released and relented, you now cleverly adapted and reinvented, you see your life is a great and wonderful gift, expressing a greater passion and intensity, taking charge and making choices decisively with the skill of a master, in things both complex and simple.

You trust in the simple yet reality that the very best way to control, is to relax and flow and release control as a concept, as you now released control, you are now in control.

Your life, now your creation, more stress-free, centered and serene, accepting what needs to be seen, and dealt with, the mighty master living inside your body chooses to seize the moment, rise above, forgive, heal, release, transcending.

For the greater the challenge, the more heroic and mighty you are, you remain, and forever become, this so true, this now and forever you do, in ways, both known and unknown to you, your automatic mind, generating serenity, the ability to rise up and truly having transcended.

You love yourself, with better thoughts, better feelings, better ideas, better habits, better reactions, while you're awake, while you are asleep, even when you dream, almost as if, someone from deep, deep inside of you, has reset a switch, a dial, or a computer, or thermostat, of some kind, all this now, both in ways instantaneous and automatic, all of your very best, all this now your very own.

Fearless Flying - 1

Relax, relax, relax. And as you relax, you allow a new, healthier and better choice in your life to take place, a potent and powerful choice to successfully take place, a brand new and completely unstoppable shift in thought, feeling, and emotion, that allows a marked improvement, an unstoppable breakthrough, right here and right now, only getting more effective and easier at each and every heartbeat and breath.

A brand new day has dawned in your life, almost like first being born, a true brand new beginning, a day where you the rise up to become and heroic and even mighty.

A new day where you can take a plane anywhere at anytime and still feel relaxed, peaceful, safe, while trusting in life, and powerfully serene and calm, and this only gets better and easier each and every day and night.

You've simply taken the pressure off, decided to relax, and enjoy the ride, so comfortable, so tired, even falling asleep.

In this moment of deep and powerful relaxation, you have come to truly recognize, embrace, and forever trust in a new truth: you are realizing and living from the idea that flying is absolutely and truly the safest form of transportation available in the world today.

Your correct response to any and all stress is to breathe deep, feel like you are being bathed in a sea of tranquility and protection, relax, trust and profoundly rise above.

You truly come to realize, today planes are better maintained, flight crews are better trained, more efficient and all of the ground support structures like radar and air traffic control are state of the art, utilizing all of the most modern and safest equipment. In fact, flying is safer than riding in a car or walking down street in many cases.

So right now, whether or not you realize it or not, in the very best of ways, ways both unknown or even unknown to you, your mind is making powerful and permanent choices from deep, deep inside of you, a powerful shift in consciousness that you are safe, you are protected, you are trusting, you are now choosing to be calm, you are now profoundly choosing to upgrade your thinking and right now and whenever needed, you are even upgrading your ways of feeling, powerfully supporting yourself and feeling safe, protected and taken care of, flying and planes, your new friends.

As you relax, easily, beyond limits, your effective powerful, dynamic and always successful subconscious mind is working away, now creatively and effectively in your favor, supportive ways that protect you and take better care of you, even heroically, as you relax deeper and further, beyond any and all former barriers from now done, shunted into the past and absolutely and forever resolved, grown up beyond, now and forever finished and done chapters of your life, making and creating new, happier, healthier, completely supportive, better choices.

You have chosen to correctly respond to any stress, any and all formerly disturbing thoughts or feelings in your new correct manner, by choosing to powerfully trust and dynamically relax through any and all stress, just letting it all go.

You've even come up with a new way to beat any and all stress and any and all tension, by correctly choosing to relax, by always remembering to deep breathe your way into relaxation, in fact, you are always aware, that your easiest, most potent and powerful way to relax, is to deep breathe, slow and steady deep, deep relaxation breath, now feeling centered, trusting, and profoundly protected, which always allows you to relax all of your body, all of your emotions, all of your mind, and even all of your spirit, harmoniously relaxing you all over.

You have chosen correctly to let go of and relax far, far away from any and all old worries from the past, choosing instead to be happy, calm and powerful.

All of those old useless, unwanted, unneeded, irrational, even silly childish worries and all of their negative energy are going, going, gone, just because that's what you've chosen powerfully and correctly to do.

As you have moved on from the ways of childhood, so too, your uncomfortable past released and now knowing a better harmonious balance is now yours!

And it's so easy for you. Even now, maybe even without noticing, you are just letting all of these past experiences, just gone, almost like how you can forget a dream after just a few moments after you awaken.

You are just willing to forget and let go of your unwarranted and unnecessary fears, and all of their past influence upon you, they are getting harder to remember, harder to think about, more comfortable, just moving on, having lost all of their past influence upon you, just drifting and floating away, forgetfully away, so very comfortably far, far away from you.

You can actually feel those useless and negative energies just lifting up, off and far, far away from you. Less and less important are those old and destructive energies and fears, released and forgiven, more and more powerful you are and you remain, vigilant, dynamically thriving beyond doubts and fears, wherever they might be coming from or wherever they might be or whatever they are.

A powerful new feeling is emerging in place of your old feelings, inner strength, inner wisdom, inner knowing, inner serenity, feeling all of those energies supporting you profoundly; what you knew of these, what you felt of these, you now know, feel and are protected by.

The part of you that has always gotten through, the part of you that always succeeds, the part of you that has thrived, been victorious, the part of you that knows doubtlessness, the part of you that knows fearlessness and the part of you that knows harmony and all the energy of all of your past moments of this kind of success is adaptively and powerfully embracing all that you are and is upon you now, forever flourishing.

As you just know, very powerfully, from deep, deep inside, that all of you has been inspired, upgraded, improved changed, protected, taken care of, so you now, a real, true and mighty master of your life, thoughts and feelings, right now seizing all moments to be better, to be mighty, to rise above, to thrive, succeed and flourish, vanquishing the childish distrust of the past, all of this becoming so very easy for you to do.

You now mighty and easily rising up to thrive and succeed at any and all challenges in your life, master and hero of your world, vanquishing victim-hood thinking and replacing it as you trust in life, your life and all of your existence, as your inner wisdom supports you unbeatably as well as all of those around you.

Now and you can feel your inner wisdom and courage surfacing as you relax, deeper and deeper, relaxing beyond any and all former barriers, truly redefined: relaxing and trusting, relaxing and powerful, relaxing and mighty, relaxing and heroic, calm and smiling inside, all of this getting easier and more dynamic, more effectively adaptive, more supportive and profound, redefining you and unlimiting you, successfully triumphant, each and every time you enjoyably repeat this exercise on your own, blockages from your now and forever done, previous chapters of your life, now less and less meaningful to you, dissolving easily and forever away.

You now, even further along and more successfully and effectively improved than even you had imagined. You know, it's really like you've done 3, 6, 9 years worth of healing and moving forward in your mind in this regard right now, and more, each and every time you enjoy this process on your own, almost like someone from deep, deep inside of you has reset a switch, a dial, a powerful and life changing computer of some kind, released a valve which drains away upset or imbalance, or even adjusted a thermostat of some kind, easily allowing you to succeed and thrive here, or instead just successfully break through.

It's truly amazing, how powerful a little relaxation can be, as you have now relaxed beyond past disharmonies, into a new harmony, more mighty, more fearless and forever freed! It feels great to be so free.

Whatever the challenge, however you might be challenged, you are rising above, slow and steady, deep and soothing breath balancing you and heroically guiding you, breaking you through here, guiding your way, you glowingly make the most of things, an inspiration to those around you, whether it's turbulence, air pockets, bad weather, or anything else, for the greater the past challenge, the even greater you now remaining serene and above it all.

By now forever releasing the past and old thoughts and feelings that once ever stood in your way, you are now undeniably free and safe, every time you nod your head, you know this to be more and more true, a true and active, real part of you.

You truly know, you are empowered in these new future moments of your life! I even wonder if you can truly yet recognize, how powerful you really are and that by deep breathing slow and steady powerful life changing relaxation breath.

You are vitalizing yourself, giving yourself a very potent and most powerful gift, the gift of being able to relax your way through anything and everything in your life, into brilliant and powerfully supportive vistas, a new day has dawned in your life, not because I say so, because you have, whether or not you realize it as yet, or not, but it is happening and has happened all around you and it feels great to be so free, most especially taking a trip on a plane, something you now look forward to with a powerful, thriving happy anticipation.

This happy positive anticipation stays with you, in all moments before, during and after your trip, because you've just let the past go triumphantly and you've actually begun a brand new happier chapter of your life, which just gets better and better, even in the most surprising and supportive of heroic of ways, the very best relaxation, deep and profound.

You realize, you even notice and powerfully recognize, that you are almost feeling happier and happier, beginning right now and for the rest of your life. The best way to control, is not to control but better, to let go, flow and fly, becoming safe, trusting and free.

As you relax deeply and profoundly, you realize, you even notice and powerfully and deeply recognize, that you are almost feeling happier and happier, almost as if a happy even silly song is going through your head, just the kind of a song that would light up your heart, and make anyone who heard it, smile, laugh and feel warmed by this song, your song's happy embrace.

This gentle song allows you to smile, and release any and all tension, release and vanquish stress, in the most amazing, potent and beneficial of ways, because you are now truly free and supported and adaptively effective, in a new chapter of your life, trusting and free, supported by life and your all of your thoughts, and supportive feelings, all working effectively in your favor, empowered, mightier than any and all challenges.

Congratulations, you relax and you win, thrive and succeed here, in a brand new chapter of your life, released and freed, truly amazing and impressing everyone, most especially you.

Each and every day and night, your courage, strength, unstoppable, highly effective and adaptable determination are a powerful and motivating inspiration to both men, women and children alike, you win, as never before!

Fearless Flying - 2

You relax beyond any and all former limits into your life, trusting in your life, and within the consistency of your livelihood and life as it has always been, now only getting clearer and just better and better.

Just as each and every day, and each and every night has protected you, practically divinely guided, more certain, serene, and sure of yourself, and any other time before, because in this vital moment, at this pivotal time, you have entered into a brand new chapter of your life, where you are more protected and unbeatable than ever before. You begin to truly recognize some places deep, deep inside of you, the best way to control, is to not control, but to relax and go with the flow that is your life, and you come to astoundingly approve of and trust this fact, unbeatably as a new, more stable foundation within your life is strengthening you.

For the greater the challenge, the mightier, self-assured and more relaxed you become. All of this is just happening to you, any and all things once considered problems, are now challenges, to be stepped up to, and faced down, while looking squarely in the eye of, and now easily overwhelmed by you, as they are and they remain forever.

You are succeeding at anything easily and most effectively, feeling totally powerful as you rise up to do this. It is almost as if someone from deep, deep inside of you has reset a switch, the dial, a thermostat, or a computer of some kind, easily strengthening you, dynamically motivating you, shaking off any and all now done former imbalances, generating balance, while you step forward mightily and boldly into your life.

All areas of your life now more overwhelmingly affected by your strength, your self compassion, and your ability to transcend now done, finished and vanquished former limits, from your now old, previous and now finished chapters of your life. Any and all challenges now done, you have effectively reversed and vanquished that energy back upon itself, as you a liberated, safe, serene and sure of yourself.

Whenever you have to fly soon, you are happily motivated now by the adventure of what you are going to deal with, not because I say so, but because it is now the nature of your own unlimiting and dynamic mind to break through here unbeatably, and so it is, and so it remains forever.

You now upgrade your serenity, and the fact, that you will remain active and free, even Divinely protected, trusting in a stronger sense of yourself and your life, and the actual real and true protection Divinity is offering you in the reality of your life.

You recognize the safety and even the safety statistics, finding even clever ways of trusting in those facts. You relax and recognize the physics of how all of this works, and how that which is real remains unthreatened and strong, yielding yet safe, while that which is unreal does not exist, most especially fears from previous and now finished chapters of your life right now.

You're feeling safe, liberated and sure of yourself, trusting in your life as well as in all that you are. Any and all of this becoming easier and better for you in the most profound of ways.

In this new and reset chapter of your life, each and every aspect of flying makes you feel calm, adventurous, happy, self-loving, protected, with cool gentle skin, and your calm and soothing heart rate, your relaxed and peaceful stomach, your deep and soothing breath guides your way into a pleasant experience, even into a place where you can relax and sleep as needed.

Any and all of this becoming easier and better over time, regardless of the challenge, For the mightier the challenge, the more relaxed and confident you become. So whether it's anticipating a flight, you know to use deep breathing, creating a balanced and calm stomach, a relaxed, soothing heart rate, a better you, breaking through, unbeatable. I wonder if you yet completely realize, how truly easy this is for you, any and all of this, becoming easier and better for you.

In any and all places where you once got nervous, you now become even more cleverly effective and adaptive while remaining calm, centered and balanced. Any and all of this getting easier and more profoundly effective overtime. For within yourself now and always, you are as free as you need to be from deep inside of you.

You now in every aspect of your life, more free and in control than ever before, loving yourself enough to relax and to go with the flow, and like a mighty river running down the side of a mountain in the spring, you flow over, around through and beyond any and all former and now done obstacles from previous chapters in your life, as you truly know a foundational difference has taken place within your life, your heart, your stomach, your skin, and your mind, all now comfortable and supportive, completely recalibrated and reset in your favor, to reveal a greater truth, a better presence, a better life, a better experience as well as a better you.

Just as with any other time in your life when you've broken though unbeatably, so too now this time, you do and it's easy and more so powerful, long-lasting and getting easier over time.

Fearless Flying – 3

You relax and you trust in your life, each and every day has supported you, each and every night has taken care of you very well, and as a deep and powerful personal truth, from levels deep within you foundationally, you begin to recognize and even realize, or simply even just now know, the best way to control anything is to relax through any and all self-imposed barriers, become serenely forever freed.

Easily now, remaining free of any sort of feelings or desires for controlling, flowing without frustration, flowing frustration-free, relaxing and releasing, allowing true control within yourself to take place, and you are now and forever freed, feeling a new sense of trust in your life, internal as well as external support.

Far or nearby, close or far away, high or low, you relax and release, instantly generating a feeling of soothing, calming, warm hearted life support, as your muscles relax, and you even feel sleepy, so very easily and effectively able to relax and even sleep and rest while traveling on a plane anywhere.

Having entered an unstoppable brand new chapter of your life, you relax and completely, just totally trust in the flow of your life, almost as if someone from deep, deep inside of you, has opened a valve and released any and all old discomforts, from the past clearing you, cleansing you, cleaning you, uplifting you, restoring you, and making you mightier than any challenge presented in your life, truly, just it has always been, all things in harmony and in balance, and now restoring you completely, you rise up, in relaxed and comfortable strength, even heroically, breaking through here unbeatably.

Your mind now relaxed anytime you get on a plane, your body temperature comfortable, your breath slow and soothing, your heart rate, comfortable, slow and steady, love for yourself and life supporting.

You have decided to move into a brand new chapter, while traveling on planes, you are calm, unafraid, you relax a deeper and further now, and recognize that deeply releasing any and all discomforting energy and thought, allows now you to feel more comfortable, releasing stress and strain.

You are now in a brand new chapter, having grown up a little bit more, free from the past, and more certain and serene than ever before, not because I say so, but because it is the advantage now of your own mind and passionate spirit to do this.

As your mighty inner hero, now unblocks you and moves you out of your own way, shinning a new light onto and liberating you from forever, any and all old shadows, bringing forth happy success sensations for all that you are in each and every moment, certain and sure.

Especially whenever most challenged, you move into your own world, easily able to thrive and succeed, in ways both known and unknown to you, while you were awake, while you're asleep, even while you floating and dreaming into a peaceful night of sleep, you relaxing and life supporting dreams, working these issues out within ways both known and unknown to you, achieving unbeatable success here.

Ahh, it feels great to be so free, calm, and relaxed, while knowing and living a better, more self-respecting, effective truth.

Any and all of this now becoming a permanent part of whoever you are and are growing into, free, free at long last, it feels great to be so free, trusting in your life, lighter, and light-hearted, liberated, dynamic, able, sitting on a plane, making you want to rest, relax, trust, and sleep, awakening at your destination, happy, calm, and excited in a beneficial, happy way to be there.

Like every other trip you've taken already, you arrive safely, and based on your years of experience, knowing the real and lasting life fulfilling truth now, life just taking care of you, free of now vanquished childish fears, strong and powerful as an adult, now and shall forever be.

Any and all things, images, sensations, noises, feelings, actions, reactions, now are recalibrated and reset to allow greater concentration and deeper and more soothing relaxation, all things working in your favor to break you through here.

For the greater any challenge, the greater any stress, the more soothing and deep your breathing, the more calm your thoughts and you, or just even your reactions and feelings, and your regular comfortable heartbeat, the more comfortable your skin, the greater your ability to rise above and breakthrough, by relaxing through the barriers of the past, open wide, safe and free as you are now firmly and steadily in a brand new chapter of your life, choosing to thrive and succeed, really rising above, having broken through.

Any and all of your internal and external systems, now reprogrammed in your favor as you step forward and advance, forever freed, more real and true to you, each and every time you smile, blink, or shake your head yes or no, all of your abilities to thrive, more truly known and affirmed.

All that you are, your body, your emotions, your mind, your imagination, embraced by the coordinating and harmonious oneness of your mindful and life-affirming spirit, all work together in concert, to break you through, as the release of old and now going and gone, unpleasantness, discomfort, and any heaviness of the past, now lifted up and off, far, far away from you, you feel a release, you are released, you know this to be true.

All of you now knowing a higher truth, as anything you put your mind to, now more easily than ever before within your grasp.

Heroically freed, you now venture ever onward to seize your success and make it one with you, making success yours, while enjoying feelings of satisfaction and success, as a deep and true part of you now knows this and makes this all your very own.

Having done all of the necessary work, succeeding brilliantly. The truth real, this is yours, certain and sure.

Overcoming a Fear of Being Viewed, Blush Response

As you relax, and float, and drift, and dream, you find your ability to reset, recalibrate, and rebalance yourself, most especially whenever challenged in any way at all, more coalesced, more focused, more easily and effectively adaptable, more instantaneously and dynamically triggered, effective and working, than any reactions that ever once stood in your way.

From this moment now you are in a brand new chapter of your life, thriving and succeeding, breaking through. Your correct response to any and all challenges from previous chapters of your life, which are now and forever done, is to deep breathe, relax, feel better, and know that you are meant to be there, and it really is okay and fine, just being you.

For regardless of who is seeing you, you're feeling safe, centered, and serene, okay, just fine and good, your skin is cool to the touch, and in perfect balance for you, for things from the past that once stood in your way are now more easily under your control, each and every day, each and every night, all of this is getting better and better, each and every breath, each and every heartbeat, all of this is just getting better and better.

In order to flow and to move beyond, you are giving yourself permission to be nervous, but instead, responding automatically by deep breathing, relaxing beyond all the barriers, into a brand new chapter of your life, and then choosing to do something better for yourself, not because I say so, but because it is the nature of your own mind, your ability to transcend, to rise above, and to become all mighty.

In this moment of deep and true profound relaxation, you are activating your mighty inner hero, the part of you that is doubtless and fearless, the part of you that would be able to save children from great danger like a fire, to now working in your favor, cleverly, adaptively, and unbeatably.

For the greater the challenge is, the greater your inner hero is at reversing that energy back upon itself, skillfully, effectively adaptively, flowing ever onward into a brand new chapter of your life, feeling confident, calm, safe and serene.

For any and all of the things that warmed up your skin emotionally, are now more easily under your control, almost as if in these few powerfully and truly life changing moments, you have done 4, 9, 16 or even 22 years worth of healing.

Almost as if someone from deep, deep inside of you, has reset permanently, adaptively, effectively, and has forever reset a switch, a dial, a computer, or turned down your thermostat, to work effectively in your favor, effortlessly and effectively.

In fact truly, you are making peace with other people's need to view you, as your self-confidence, drive, determination and self-esteem seem to be gently lifting and rising going higher and higher, filling you up with confidence and strength.

For whatever the focus of others are or might be, both real or imagined, your focus is serenity on all levels of your being, physically, emotionally, mentally, spiritually, as a new harmony of peace, tranquility, gentleness, ease, forgiveness, self-respect, self-esteem, and building self-confidence now embraces all that you are.

Foundationally re-focused and structurally grounded, you are and you remain, forever forgiven, healed and released, into the very best of a supportive and more comfortable way of living and experiencing your life ahead.

As you now relax beyond any and all barriers, further and further with each and every breath and heartbeat, even 85,000 times deeper and further each and every breath, each and every heartbeat, each and every word that you hear, you are in fact either releasing, or maybe just forgiving and just letting go of any and all blockages, any and all judgments, any and all thoughts and feelings, that once ever triggered uncomfortable reactions within your body or your mind, both known and unknown to you.

You have simply moved forward, stepped forward and set yourself free, stepping forth into a brand new chapter of your life, okay to view and be viewed, at one with yourself and at peace with all things and people.

Generating greater self respect, self-appreciation, your connection with other people now instead warms your heart and your mind, as each slow and steady deep breath guides your way. In fact, all of your reactions are now recalibrated and reset in your favor unstoppably in ways both known and unknown to you, in ways most clever, workable, effective and adaptive.

It just feels great to be so free and liberated, safe in your zone, as you're always working in your favor, your clever and reactively adaptive mind is now working with you, whether you realize it or not, in ways to generate the greatest profound affect and improvement in your life unbeatably, unstoppably, even heroically.

Weather out in public, or at work, in fact anyplace, you are released, relaxed and comfortable, truly, you now deeply know, you are relaxing beyond any and all barriers, willing to be limitless, seizing this profound moment in which to heal, reorganized, regenerate, seizing all profound moments of healing, and making all of this your very own, feeling the embrace of this success and support right here and right now.

It has been said that in my vulnerability lies our greatest strength, and there is no need to be defensive, as you accept a more open to role and outlook on life, experiences, as you have now decided to explain and educate, rather than to defend, rather than receive an impact, you redirect all reactions and energies, flow and succeed, even if surprised in some way, you're looking forward to greater challenges, because you are in a new place in your life, mighty and heroically breaking through.

You are so very free of ever second guessing yourself, any action, any thought, any word, any construct of language, you are just doing fine. Free of over-analyzing or second guessing, even your dream state is allowing pleasant dreams that allow you to usher in a brand new chapter of your life, free of overreacting and in fact fearless and mighty.

It's almost as if the entire world is now working to support you, and encouraging you and cheering you on, ushering in your success unbeatably, they want what's best for you. You generate it and create it, trusting in the life you create, manifesting and creating profound improvement in your life right now.

You are now serene and certain, foundationally recalibrated, upbeat and looking forward to your life, whether off to the side or the center of attention. You are better than okay, and you are doing better and better, as you have made a new choice for a better day, a better night, a better life.

Skillfully adapting and improving, each little step forward means a lot, and soon you're miles and even light years beyond challenges from now done previous chapters of your life, free at long last, you look forward to each and every day doing better and better, as all of this and any of this, becomes easier and easier.

Stress Management - Feeling Relaxed During Medical Testing Procedures

As you relax deeper and further, it occurs to you that you have relaxed your way beyond any and all former barriers from the now finished past, into a brand new more stress-free chapter of your life.

As you relax even deeper and further, it is almost as if someone from deep, deep inside of you has reset a switch, turned the dial, reset a thermostat, released a valve, or activated a powerful computer of some kind which allows you to instantly and powerfully breakthrough, more self-supporting and effective, to the highest and greatest good for you and those you love most, most especially yourself.

Any and all things that once stressed you out involving any sort of medical treatment, review or exam, you now more easily take in stride knowing and feeling this from deep inside.

Your best response and more immediate reaction to any situation you once felt to be distressing is to relax your way deeply and comfortably, melting away any and all stress from your body, until you are, by slow and steady breath, assured that you are and you remain stress-free, calm and relaxed.

Your breathing and heart rate, slow, deep, and rhythmic, instantly alleviating and releasing any and all now done former anxiety or stress, completely freed now, in ways both known and unknown to you, as your automatic mind, now so fine-tuned, so reset, so recalibrated, to allow you a completely noticeable breakthrough and serene success here, as you succeed with the skill of a master at this.

For the greater the challenge, the more relaxed and mightier you become, even heroic.

Any and all things that ever once stressed you out, including medical tests or procedures or other situations, you now relax beyond while finding tranquility, ease, peace and moreover, deepest serenity within yourself that now seems to keep you unmistakably calm, or maybe just seems to bubble up to the surface keeping you calm and relaxed.

Your heartbeat slow and steady, you at a different yet better serene and peaceful centered pace, your breathing slow and rhythmic, your body now under your calming control, to allow you peace, ease, tranquility and trust In the care and professionalism of those around you, and truly the process of life itself.

The very best way to control, to relax and trust, trust in the flow of life and the process. for the greater the challenge, the mightier you become, in tranquility and inner and outer peace as well.

It is almost like whenever they go to test your body or mind in any way, whether to collect a sample of some kind, or even a simple blood pressure test, you become so calm, so very relaxed, so comfortably at peace, so still, so tranquil, thinking of pleasant, happy memories and feelings from the past, while almost completely re-experiencing that happiness, ease, comfort and joy.

Almost as if it's calming, soothing, comforting, energy blanket of restoration, ease, tranquility, peace, and support, beyond what even those words mean, re-experiencing their feelings, sensing this, feeling this, knowing this, responding to this in ways most appropriate and most clearly, completely effective, automatically generated, in ways most effective, just for you.

All of this begins to just happen on its own, as your automatic mind, your dynamic eternal wise mind, is now working this out in ways both known and unknown to you for your greatest benefit possible, and so it is, and so it comfortably remains forever, in ways most joyous, self-loving, self improving, and beneficial just for you begins to happen automatically on their own, effortlessly, with highest and most complete dynamic results and experience for you.

Almost like memorizing this feeling of relaxation as a safe, happy place to be and you more easily able to bring yourself back here most especially whenever challenged.

It is almost like past imbalances, whether they were emotional, mental, or any kind of imbalance, have now been washed clean from you, as you are now more sure than ever that you are cleansed, healed, and restored, in ways most effective and complete, on each and every breath, on each and every heartbeat.

Relaxed and calm blood flow, supported and embraced by the environment and the people around you, now more comfortable, certain, serene, and sure, that you have risen to a mightier, better, effective, results-oriented for success and breakthrough place.

A place in a brand new and better chapter of your life, succeeding here, knowing any and all of this to be true and sure, as your dynamic mind is now working this out to greatest and maximum best potential benefit to you completely, in body, emotions, mind, even spirit, generating highest and greatest harmony and calm and soothing strength.

You serene strength renewed, as your body under any testing condition now more relaxed, meltingly calm and at complete rest and peace, now more calm, now more complete, now more whole, now more reconditioned and rejuvenated to relax and make your way through, flowing ever onward to test excellence, calmness and best results possible.

Driving Free of Fear

As you relax, and float, and dream, while feeling deeply relaxed, a true sense of soothing calmness, and absolutely wonderful, a new thought begins to arise in your mind, a knowing and glowing thought, that truly, you have entered a brand new chapter of your life, feeling mightier and more adaptive, more easily able to rise above and fully and forever transcend, all of the things that ever once stood in your way.

In this new chapter of your life, you have made deep and profound adjustments and improvements, recognizing these improvements, and making them your very own. Your correct response to any and all situations that once ever caused you any kind of stress, is to relax, taking deep and slow, steady breath, as you feel, sense and truly now are able to generate when necessary and only know the embrace of, a more stress-free, and relaxed you.

As you begin to breathe slowly and deeply, there is a shift in the energy within your body, feeling and knowing this improvement, as what once was the may have felt like nervousness, is now a sense of serenity, and peace, harmony and balance, centeredness and calm strength, yet profound relaxed determination, that allows you to move forward in your life, and allows you to mightily and easily create a calm and serene you, a calm and serene experience which is your life.

Whatever may come, you trust in the fact, a powerful and directed calm, and serene focus, guides you from what once was darkness and shadow, to a place of joyously inspired, divinely guided light, a sense of purpose, a sense of direction, that allows you to mightily transcended any and all former limits, which are now and forever done and finished, in this brand new chapter of your life.

For the mightier than challenge once was, the greater and mightier you become, reaching higher, rising higher. As you relax even deeper now, all the way down, you also relaxing beyond all former limits, and barriers, in your life, into a place of serenity and strength, a foundation home base, allowing yourself to breakthrough here, unstoppably, as you now know this to be in fact true, which is spreading adaptively, working effectively, and allowing you to feel and truly become unstoppable, whenever it is you need to drive anywhere, locally or whether on a highway, over a bridge, or a tunnel, whether driving a long distance or short one, you are in your zone, both aware, clear, calm and focused, and just doing better.

You know, it's almost like someone from deep, deep inside of you, has easily and forever effectively, reset a switch, a dial, a computer, or a thermostat of some kind, which has drained off any and all unneeded, undeserved, unwelcome, fear from the past, while centering you and focusing you, knowing what the pros know, how they drive, you drive, what they know, you know, where they look, you look, how they maintain safety, you maintain safety, how they react, you react, how they adapt, you adapt.

And therefore you in fact do, calmly, peacefully, effectively, dynamically, relaxing and trusting, while achieving any and all desired goals and beneficial outcomes. Any and all of this is becoming substantially more and more profound, easier and better for you, more dynamic, more adaptive, more clear, as you visualize now and easily achieve successful breakthrough outcomes. Not because I say so, because you have decided this and so it is.

You may even be laughing from deep inside, feeling so triumphant, so victorious, so skillfully adaptive, that you are breaking through here and succeeding, almost as if in this moment, or in any and all moments of reinforcement, with even greater and more profound outcomes, you even imagine or perhaps know from deep, deep inside, you have done twelve to fourteen years worth of healing on this, in just a few moments.

Like a child staying within the lines of a coloring book, you are guided, you drive, you signal, maintain safety. You begin to realize how in fact easy it is, just like it used to be, but now only better, to drive on a highway, while skillfully paying attention to the rules of the road, so subconscious, automatic and so second nature, that you even begin to look forward to driving, and even long distance driving, for you are and you remain so very inspired, and recalibrated, that you love to face down all challenges from now previous chapters of your life, now done, and now moved on from, looking forward actually to driving places while trusting in your life, and in divine protection.

For in these moments of relaxation, inspiration, and recalibration, you truly feel great, so mighty, fearless, dynamic, ready to look into the eye of and easily face down any and all challenges that have the one stood in your way, out of your way now faced down, truly knowing this to be in fact, you are unbeatable.

This new you, courageous and audacious, dynamic, mighty and creative, trusting, dynamic, is in fact, free and rising to the top, allowing you to become in forever remain, calm, while giving yourself a break in all thoughts, emotions and reactions, feeling more trusting and more self loving, tranquil, peaceful, cool, calm, serene, relaxing beyond any and all limits into a greater and better truth, completely sensitive and unruffled, driving skillfully and peacefully while remaining forever and anger free, free of rage, treating yourself in a better and more loving fashion.

In fact truly, your correct response, to any challenge in your life, is to allow deep and soothing patterns of breath, in slowly, held for a moment or so, and released even more slowly to automatically kick in, and takeover, generating serenity and inner as well as outer peace. Your new and improved, correct reaction to any and all challenges, is deep and steady breathing, while relaxing and becoming adaptive and inspired to break through unbeatably.

Almost like some cloudy energy that's once been around you has been removed making you feel wonderful, as a new energy has replaced it that now inspires you, gives you strength, guidance, adaptability, a calm and soothing heartbeat, comfortable skin, and deep soothing breath. Your thoughts, your emotions, your mind, your feelings, your body, the energy all around your head, allows for calm and serene powerful focus and success here.

Each and every night while you sleep through the night peacefully and are more easily able to fall back to sleep whatever you need to, in the comfort of a bed that supports your relaxation and rejuvenation, and body wonderfully and restfully, as now even your dreams, peacefully adjust your thoughts and feelings to allow ultimate success here, while forgiving, healing, and releasing, any and all imbalances, and uncomfortable experiences wherever they came from, whether known or unknown to you, powerfully and unstoppably beginning this brand new chapter of your life.

You now allow yourself forever to feel wonderful here. Deep breathing generates inner peace and calmness, a true and correct trust in life, and a better you, which now unstoppably surfaces, as the world around you supports this better you, and a brilliant new you in a new and improved chapter of your life.

More easily able to achieve all desired outcomes, amazing and impressing everyone, most especially yourself! Your success is its own reward as you are more easily able to drive, shop, meet friends, and instinctively operate your vehicle safely and correctly while, checking your mirrors every few seconds, signaling, allowing safety distance around you, focused on the road, driving skillfully from years of experience, and active and reacting as necessary while focused on your driving as well as those around you.

You're doing any and all of this, just like years ago, only better this time, while adaptively, skillfully, and cleverly knowing this from deep inside of you as profound and foundational truth within your life. Just like any other time in your life, when you were challenged and had to do something, thriving in spite of the situation to get it done, you now do, knowing that you are now fulfilled and doing just fine.

Whether nearby or far away, you are determined, and clever, doing just fine and feeling better. You have made up your now reconditioned and supportive mind, fully liberating yourself and your life with the embrace in this new and profound truth. Any and all of this, achieved, not because I say so, because that's the nature of your own mind, body, spirit to do this, and so this is your new life.

And so it just is, and forever remains, smiling from deep inside, you now just doing better and better, while remaining a very upbeat, outgoing person, glowing both in heart and mind, glowing inside and out, smiling and appreciating every moment of your life, heroically facing down any and all challenges, for the mightier the challenge, the better you are.

Driving Fears: Bridges, Elevated Roadways, Panic

Your automatic and always working in your favor, dynamic, breakthrough subconscious mind is now working in ways known and unknown to you, correcting any and all unpleasantness and imbalances, generating in their place clarity, calmness, focus, pleasantness, balance, harmony, mighty, talent, will expand in your ability to transcend any and all now done past chapters of your life,.

Deep inside you know this to be true, you know this to be best, it is real to you more and more each and every day and night.

Your correct response to each and every anything, known or unknown to you, that once caused unpleasantness or upset, is to start taking slow and steady deep, deep soothing, stilling, calming, peaceful, centering breaths, which allows you to create serenity, centeredness, as foundationally powerful waves of inner peace begin flowing from heart and mind all around and through you, calming you and restoring you instantly.

I wonder if you even yet realize how automatic and truly powerful this transforming experience is going to feel, sense it all around you in your life.

Smiling from places deepest and true from the core of your being, this not only becomes more real and true, but a real known true fact you and your life as a brand new chapter of your life is now forever begun.

You begin to realize that driving on a road means driving in the lane, and driving and aligning your driving as the road goes straight or turns, stop or go.

Regardless of the structure, a road is a road, whether the road be a flat road somewhere in the country, long and straight, twisting or turning, whether that road be somewhere in a suburb, a side street, whether the road is contained within a city, or on a highway, bridge or a tunnel, all roads are pretty much the same.

Like a coloring book, the idea is to stay between the lines, in a lane, drive safely checking your mirrors and the environment around you, following traffic laws, regardless if it is over a bridge, or a low road, whether it is an elevated road or the highway, you remain clear, supported by yourself, as your mighty inner hero, is now rising to the top, to support you.

Allow yourself to feel mighty, keep alert and focused, while you are now more in tune with your body, and mind, even emotions, any and all supportive feelings, to keep you clear and alert, to know when you are tired and should pull over and rest,.

A sense of all that is going around you now ever more acute and focused, almost intuitive and from on high, while controlling your vehicle, the skill of your many years of driving and experience, even training, and insight from others, will remain clear and sharp, focused and clear, almost as if every where you drive is like a local street, easily and forever getting the job done.

Your automatic mind now ceaselessly working from places of greatest importance and impact, as you remain so cool and clear, vanquishing and alleviating any and all loose ends that ever once stood in your way, almost like a giant burden has been lifted from you.

Ahhhhhh, it feels so good as you break through here, calm and cool, clear and free.

Almost as if someone from the deepest places inside of you has reset a switch, a dial, a thermostat, or a computer of some kind, resetting you, recalibrating you, restoring you, activating you in ways completely appropriate and absolutely effective, dynamically and heroically here, now, always, and forever, you are certain and sure, you have broken through here, all issues resolving themselves for you, automatically.

Anything and everything that once caused you upset , or imbalance, those things vanquished themselves.

You now liberated safe and forever stronger, fluid, adaptive, and cutting yourself a break, in ways both known and unknown to you, as slow and steady breaths and soothing, comfortable, life affirming, inspirational heartbeats, guide your way brightly to a better day, and a more restful safer and more comfortable night.

From here on out, you are now and forever restored, safe, heroic, and liberated certainly ever sure, in this new chapter of your life, safe and strong, fluid and adaptive.

Your mind now working out cleverly any and all of the very best results to breaking through here and so it is, and so remains forever.

ThunderStorm – Overcoming Fear (Child)

As you relax, float, drift and dream, you get an idea and begin to remember something.

You always knew that as you grew up bigger in your life into a young [man, woman] or into a full sized [man, woman], that any and all fears about the weather would not be a part of your life, no longer be important.

So as you relax, float, drift, and dream, you now realize that you have grown up just a little bit more, maybe five or six or seven years worth more grown up, where uncomfortable feelings about the weather are now being released, healed, forgiven, let go of...

And instead, you are the strong one, the mighty one, the one who relaxes, taking calming and soothing, slow, steady deep breaths, slow and steady breaths, feeling stronger by relaxing.

The correct way for you to feel, as you now are strong, powerful, heroic, more grown up, the way to react, the way for you to behave, your best choice, is to take slow and steady breaths, and as you do your entire body calms down.

Every thought and every feeling becomes stronger and better, taking so much better care of you, you are powerful, happy and free, almost like the best holiday ever, your best birthday, happy, happy heart, a smile on your face, more grown up, a bigger grownup, and just as you are no longer interested in things that once interested a little kid, you are now so much more interested in feeling better about yourself and your life.

So too now, you have released and let go of, any nervousness about weather, clouds, rain, thunder, because you are more grown up, and always taking better care of you, knowing that you are and will remain okay.

It is fine for you to be wet from rain, and even if it is sunny, or cloudy, wet or raining, you are now more of a man than ever before, stronger, better, more powerful, or instead maybe even just a bit more grown up, as you are forgiving, letting go of, releasing, growing up beyond, and mightier, having made the deeper and more powerful choice to feel better.

So much more of the big [boy, girl], so much more of a young [man, lady] then you ever were as a baby or a little kid.

For the more stormy the weather, the bigger, mightier and more hero like you are inside, as well as outside, most especially inside, for you, and for those you love, but mostly because you love yourself better and are doing better than ever before.

You recognize and realize, every day, and every night, that anything that shows up in your life, is something you will learn from and decide to face and deal with.

The crazier the weather, the more calm you are inside, and you now know this completely as the truth, as you are and you continue to be bigger, and mightier, than any challenge in front of you, and you are forgiving, releasing, healing, and feeling better than, anything that ever once upset you.

You're sure of this and know this to be true, not because I say so, but because that is just the way it is, becomes, and forever remains, letting go of the ways of a baby or a little kid, in ways both known and unknown to you.

So even if it is cloudy outside, you are calm, happy, and feeling fine, and determined to feel that way no matter what the weather is doing, may do, or will do.

You remember that rain makes plants and flowers grow, and cleans the earth, and it's okay with you, to do what you have to do, to relax, laugh, and feel happy inside; it's okay to feel better and happier in your life and so you figure out ways to make that happen.

If you see lightning or hear a thunderstorm, you relax completely all over, inside and out, as it maybe reminds you of fireworks on the Fourth of July, and that's okay, making you smile and laugh, choosing to feel happier and better instead.

Your correct response to rain, lightning or thunder is to be more grown up, because right now in this moment you are feeling better about yourself, almost as if from deep, deep inside of you, somebody has pushed a button making this okay, flipped a switch, making you feel fine, happier and calmed down, opened up a valve that releases any and all uncomfortable feelings.

Instead, you choose to feel happy and fine, and removing any unpleasantness far, far away from you, or almost as if someone has adjusted the thermostat, as your breathing and body temperature feel just fine, things once upsetting, now every day and every night so less important to you right now.

Overcoming a Fear of Singing in Public

Relaxing deeper and further and let your mind wander to a place of inspirational success, breakthrough, and victory - a place where you unbeatably rise above any and all now forever done, limits from previous chapters of your life, as in this moment of relaxation, you are and in fact truly relaxing and yet embraced by an energy that allows you to unbeatably flourish, in body, emotions, mind and even spirit, you are practically Divinely guided.

In this place, just imagine yourself now, at your very best, almost as if within these few brief moments of relaxation, most especially every time you repeat this wonderfully enjoyable technique on your own, you are doing the equivalent of seven to nine years worth of powerful and accelerated inner and outer healing, yielding maximum results.

You know you can actually feel this inspirational support and healing, in every fiber of your being, feeling it within your shoulders, in your breathing, in your spine, in the muscles that support your back, in your hips and in your legs, around the back of your head, your face now glowing with their radiant golden-white light of victorious breakthrough inspiration.

In this place, and in this moment, you now and forever unbeatable. Just letting your talent go, flow, and all of this becoming easier and better, singing and expressing joyously, from your heart and from your mind, generating harmony, as your powerful dynamic subconscious mind is allowing you to achieve optimal results, as any and all of this becomes as natural as tying your shoelace or walking.

You both now and forever, determined to rise above any and all challenges, and to truly have fun here.

All of this now and forever more easy and natural, whether singing with a group of people, whether singing [XX Sabbath songs at the Sabbath table, singing Happy Birthday with a group] not because I say so, but because it is time and it is so, now and forever, as your dynamic mind is working out patterns of success, and inspired breakthroughs, while you are awake, while you are asleep, even while you dream at night happily, sleeping peacefully through the night into the following day, awakening refreshed and ready to seize all moments to enjoy your life, and to share your gifts.

For the greater the resistance once was, the easier it is directed away from you, as your mighty inner hero, the part of you that is doubtless and truly powerful, has now and forever been activated from deep inside of you, and dynamically in your favor, knowing newer and greater truth, as the ability to rise above is yours now.

In this heroically inspired and polished chapter of your life, you begin to trust in your life, your choices, your desires, your inspirations, and the decisions and choices you make, which now lead to a more joyous way of life.

It is time to be happy, and whether or not it is clear to you yet, you are releasing from your life both things known and unknown to you, that no longer serve you or even once blocked you, in ways that are supportive, which will help to abundantly and limitlessly generate more supportive feelings, and inspirations, as you are now learning to love and trust yourself, even challenging yourself to do better, in this brand new and exciting chapter of your life.

In this chapter of your life, one major truth you learn to embrace, and make your very own adaptively, in ways most effective, is you are choosing to become failure free, challenge oriented, always either learning or succeeding, as those are your only options. Loving yourself now enough to cut yourself a break.

You are shining inside and out, foundationally recalibrated, reset, forgiven, healed and released, even redefined in the most loving and self-supporting ways you have ever imagined, choosing to feel wonderful instead, it feels so great to be alive.

For the only opinion that matters is yours, and as you are choosing to relax and flow beyond any and all old barriers and past moments of your life, in this new chapter of your life, more supported, carefree, and trusting of your decisions, as your inspired and creative mind, while you are awake, while you are asleep, even while you dream, generates supportive ideas, inspirations, thoughts, feelings, emotions, actions, and reactions, while generating truly better direction and focus within your life now, in knowing who you are, you now know where you stand, trusting your impressions and your instincts, ever more self-supportively, whether: [XX religiously, dating, more support of friendships and friends, career, and even where to live].

And as you relax, your mind wandering as if in a dream, coming to potent and powerful like changing insights and more limitless newer and adaptively supportive correct thoughts and feelings, so very inspired, that will take better care of you.

For beginning right now, each and every action you take, each and every reaction you have, you are choosing better and doing better, you are adaptable, focused and more determined than ever to succeed.

As you relax, you come to know all that you are doing here as the pathways and inspirations that will guide you to a better day, a better night, and a better moment in your life, living in a better moment, and realizing your dreams.

Knowing any and all of this from deep inside is a powerful truth. More certain and sure you are of this than in any of the moment in your life.

You relax, you rise and succeed here, as you now realize what you have to present and share is important.

The average person in attendance is sincerely wishing you well, wanting you to succeed, so you can sing and shine from your mind and allow all that you have to say, to share, to teach, to just flow, flowing out in a relaxed and calm, powerfully flowing fashion.

All of your thoughts and your feelings, in fact all that is your very life, supports you, in fact and in reality, all of the people who need to hear what you have to sing and share.

It's almost as if someone from deep, deep inside of you, has reset the switch, the dial, the thermostat of some kind, or even a computer which is so abundantly and deliberately effective in improving, restoring, strengthening, focusing, redirecting, all that you are into the very best place where you need to be.

As you are there, you are reconditioned into your very best. Only inspirational feelings are allowed now, and you a strengthened, for the opinions of other people matter little.

For it has been said and it has been written, "what others think of you is none of your business," - a true and powerful tenet of how you now live in this brand new chapter of your life.

Gone now and forever are the old ways, the only room you have in your life right now is for breakthrough glowing success, and so it is, so it remains.

Just imagine the embrace of now correct feelings like: confidence, self assurance, you now feeling cool and focused,. You are breathing in proper harmony and rhythm, air flowing freely, breathing from and singing from your diaphragm, relaxing and allowing all of you, to just seamlessly flow, outward - for what the pros know, you know. What they do, you do. How they respond, you respond - looking for those who are supportive, forever free of wasting time for lesser things.

You are now reconditioned and reset, so easily able to achieve any and all goals, having a new belief in yourself, but even better, true faith, that is pure and focused, but beyond faith, truly flowing into a place of divinely inspired and cared for and unbeatable knowingness.

So you are shining and sing it all, focusing upon, summoning up, and performing with only your very best talent, just like happily singing a song to a child or a group of small fascinated children.

You relax, as you allow your powerful mind to activate, all just flows out, as it should, in poised, graceful, paced, and in truly masterful ways.

The calmness that you feel right now is just exuding itself throughout your body. You are memorizing this calm and relaxed state and breathing pattern as a way to be, a way to live and a way to powerfully teach and express.

You feel the support, the understanding and appreciation of all you those who are there to share with, as your support is ever flowing, glowing, even everlasting.

And you are absolutely free to share and to express, and you are absolutely free of any and all fears. Perhaps you are even feeling fearless, or bold and courageous, in just the right form, as all of the energy of any and all past victories, breakthroughs, triumphs, and successes, that you've ever had or will have, including this moment of victories that singing has brought, are upon you now, embracing you and supporting you now, always and forever.

You are fearless and ready, free, free at last, free of everything and anything that can stand in your way, blockage free, flowing alike a mighty river down the side of large mountain in spring time, flowing over around, over and through all obstacles. You are in fact confidently feeling like an up-stoppable force, free of feeling imbalanced any way.

Free of the fear. They respect you, they need to hear from you, and they are all your biggest fans, wanting to hear all that you have to relay, completely free, you are articulate, singing with words, rhythm, and language just flowing, you are amongst friends, you are free of shaking, you are in fact composed and doing fine, cool, calm and relaxed, free of your voice trembling.

In fact, your voice is strong clear, articulate, you are in your zone, your appearance is fine, you pick 1 or 2 or 3 people to look into the eyes, easily and making friends and focused upon friends, keeping it lively, you easily gain the warm regards and best wishes of all who hear you.

You are truly and deeply and powerfully relaxed, calm and confident, with each and every slow and steady breath you take, your subconscious mind secretly but powerfully affirms this to you.

Your opinion is the only one that counts, your opinion of yourself is growing ever more positive, more beneficial, more flexible, more inspired to cut yourself a break, and you are evermore willing to thrive and to succeed.

You are ever increasingly certain of this, certain of yourself, flexible, able, calm, cool, clear, strong, with all of your very best coming easily up, unveiling even hidden talent, a great communicator emerging from deep, deep within you, almost as if, someone from deep, deep, inside of you has reset a switch, a dial, a computer, or a thermostat of some kind, easily allowing you to thrive and succeed, flow and explain, flow and express.

I wonder if you even yet realize how easy this is going to be for you, as you relax, thrive, flow and succeed?

Life Improvement: Stress Relief and Self-Forgiveness

As you release, relax, float, drift, and dream, a new and profoundly better, forgiven and released chapter of your life has now begun as your powerful, automatic and wise mind is now resetting, recalibrating, reorganizing, and returning itself to support you in the very best way is possible, both known and unknown to you.

It automatically works, free of any effort at all, to support you better, more easily able to achieve all that you desire in your life.

Your wise, automatic and dynamic mind upgrades, reinvents, restores, polishes, and improves you, activating greatest potentials into the reality that is your life around you.

More easily you forever remain able to love yourself and to do everything and anything free of expectations, simply being, to make yourself happy and healthy.

You come to a profound realization, your opinion of yourself and your thoughts about yourself, now and forever more self loving and improved, are what matter to you most.

You completely realize, recognize, what other people think of you is not your business, laughing on the inside, the realization of this so true, resonates throughout all that you are in every moment of your life.

Inside and out now reconditioned to do better and better, either easily succeeding at this, or instead just thriving.

Feeling lighter, feeling better, each and every thought, feeling, action and reaction, so much more supportive, so much more self-adapting and self-perpetuating, while allowing unbridled success for you now.

You actually begin to treat yourself the way the most ideal parent would treat the most loving child.

All the rhythms and cycles of your body reset to support you better, your breathing so much deeper and calmer, your heart rate, clear and strong, realizing and recognizing that the very best way to improve control in your life is to relax and release control, flowing ever onward into happier vistas, a forgiven and released happier and healthier better you now emerging.

Your deep and soothing now automatic breath, believes and releases anything stressful, as your active imagination and profound internal wise mind chooses serenity and peace as a way of improving and re-identifying yourself.

Your focus is on complete and limitless life improvement.

You steadfastly remain anxiety-free, stress-free, as your body is now centered, so serene, so peaceful, so balanced, so harmonized.

Now from the deepest recesses of who you are, have ever been, and shall ever be, generates self improvement as well as great potentials, even a balance of energy that triggers healing reactions within you.

Any and all of your very best now activated into the right here and now, and like a master of ancient wisdom, your wise mind guides you to take things more in stride, smiling on the inside, even greater on the outside.

Your mighty inner hero, now liberates a better day, a better way, the more soothing and tranquil night, a more rested, more improved you, as any and all of this begins to happen automatically around you, and as you notice it, you smile with pride, as highest potentials and even Divine guidance clears away and forever vanquishes any and all former shadows from now done and finish chapters of your life, it feels great to be so free.

Your perspectives elevate and improve in your favor.

In the things that matter most, as you matter more to yourself, you find clever and completely adaptive and effective ways, to allow stress and anxiety to flow around you and far, far away from you.

You are now completely ready and effectively energized, take on any and all challenges, in a calm and soothing way.

The highest healing harmony, and unconditional and adaptive strength, rising up like a mighty giant in your life, while retaining perspective, you choose to release failure and upset as concepts in your life, keeping them in perspective.

So fluid and adaptive, more serene and certain, completely ensured that a brand new chapter of your life is begun, and any and all of this is more and more real to you, more adaptive, fluid and effective, each and every time you repeat this wonderfully enjoyable technique on your own.

Even now, you have done the equivalent of fourteen to nineteen years worth of healing, as any and all of this is becoming automatically better and better, in fact, you have never been so sure of anything before ever in your life.

For in this new chapter of your life, the more mighty the challenge, the more determined you are to achieve your goals, and so it remains and forever is.

Stress Management and Setting Boundaries for Mom

In this brand new and better chapter of your life, you have decided to rise above and become mightier than any stress, by choosing instead and even better, always and automatically to relax, release, deep breathe, and become slightly detached enough from any situation, rise above it rather than being overwhelmed by it, each and every day and night, anyplace it might arise.

Rather than ever becoming a overwhelmed by stress, your automatic response to increasing stress is slower, and deeper, longer and more drawn out breath, which generates an amazing shift of energy within you, which allows you, to relax your way through any wave of stress.

It is by relaxing, and allowing just a short moment of inspiration, that you can in turn becoming empowered and inspired, and even guided, almost as if from somewhere on high, to relax and change the way you experience stress, for the mightier the stress, the mightier you become while being adaptive and fluid, clever and creative, allowing yourself inner peace.

As you relax deeper and further now, remember and re-experience the feeling of this time of tranquility and inner peace.

Feeling all around you, know its embrace, and always remember, that after just a few deep and steady soothing long breaths, you can easily bring yourself back to this place whenever you need to, whenever need be.

In a great many people's lives, stress is a factor when dealing with boundary issues.

Boundaries are established as a safety mechanism, to allow individuals self-support, self protection, and when to say enough is enough.

In this brighter, better, crisper, more inspired and empowered chapter of your life, and as a part of stress relief and stress management, you now more easily and readily are enabled to calmly and clearly express what you want, almost as if explaining to a small child, to create healing, standing up for what needs to be right, achieving easily what is necessary, what it is they need, what it is you need, and any other factor or detail, that allows you a more calm and comfortable existence.

Any and all of this happening for you automatically, and in ways most beneficial to you through the power of your automatic subconscious mind, which truly, is always working things out to your greatest benefit, even diplomatically and to the maximum benefit of all of those around you, most especially those you love, most especially you loving yourself.

For in this new chapter, the days of being overwhelmed, the nights of being overwhelmed, the moments you once experienced of being overwhelmed, are now done, releasing, healing and forgiven by you and those you now forgive once involved.

So now reset, re-tuned, recalibrated, you now, more inspired, more heroically empowered, more easily able to explain, anything and everything, which leads you, to a more tranquil and comfortable, stress-free way of life.

Whether at your job, the greater your challenge from stress, the more comfortable and free flowing, more easily able to explain, the more comfortable you are within yourself, the more easily able to draw a boundary when necessary, or to ask for more time, to complete any task necessary, now more easily able to communicate you are and you become in this way.

The more adaptive yet fortified you become, the more easily able you are to reverse the impact of stress back up on itself, liberating all that you are.

In this new chapter, you'll ask for more notice, or more time as necessary, for there is a choice, speed, or accuracy. You choose for the best.

Freer of intimidation you are and you become.

Yet the greater the challenge, the more enabled you are, to explain, to teach, to train, to set boundaries, and to teach others see it clearer and better for all involved way of getting there.

Rather then complain, you educate while standing up for yourself, in a way that enlightens all.

Rather than saying yes to everything, you bring others on board with you asking questions like, "how can we work this out in a better way together?"

In this new chapter of your life, you find that standing up for yourself, generates a greater level of respect from others, even though if at first they may not understand it.

For what others think of you, is not really any of your business, you choose instead to remain stress-free while being true to yourself.

When dealing with more personal relationships, whether your spouse or anyone else, you remain distant and detached enough during the emotional outbursts of others, removing yourself from manipulation and tantrums, and when these adults are ready to hear you, showing a better way, while speaking in positive language, which means, asking for what you want, rather than what you don't want.

Guiding, while generating better outcomes.

You have decided to remain free of ever playing that kind of manipulation game again, as often as you can, whenever and wherever and however you can.

Whatever their emotional addiction, like a rushing stream of water flowing around a boulder, you now choose to relax and become polished from the experience, as their emotions rush around you.

Other people's emotional states, you know realize the things you are unable to fix, and therefore, through your guidance when they're ready, and only when they're ready, and by your example, you more naturally find your inner leader to guide them to places of tranquility and peace by your own example , and as every time you do this, it becomes easier and better.

In this new and brighter better chapter of your life, you choose to release and remove anxiety and stress, while more solidly and completely on each and every breath and heartbeat, begin to generate more and more complete the trust in the world around you and in your life.

You now begin to realize that your life is taking good care of you, by virtue of the fact that you are here, and therefore, you know now, beyond any shadows, in the light of day you are and you remain, completely enabled to trust in your life.

You now recognize that you have enough time in your life to do everything it takes, as much time is you need, as much time as anyone else.

You trust in your life, each and every step, takes good care of you, failure free you are now and you remain, choosing instead to either succeed or learn something.

Your life is free of mistakes, simply now taken in stride as learning experiences.

Just a few minutes each and every day, just a few minutes each and every night, you plan, arrange, and make time for yourself to relax.

You truly enjoy re-experiencing relaxation and self-hypnosis, slipping into a deeper, quicker, easier, better, with greater impact results, each and every time you do this on your own.

In this new chapter of your life, while allowing yourself to play as a child once in awhile, truly, noticeably, you have grown up just a little bit more, more easily taking your life, events, people, and circumstances in stride.

By being so empowered, you become more of a shining light of guidance to other people in your world.

And yes of course you now know this to be true.

Worry is for people who do not trust. You trust, now and forever more enabled, more easily free, more easily trusting in the way your life unfolds and in the way you experience it.

In this place of rejuvenation, you allow yourself more rest, and inner and outer peace, finding a new harmony within yourself first, more easily able to balance job, family, social life and anything else in your life that is important to you, most especially your child[ren].

You take true joy in the experience of motherhood, and in the life of your child and the love that you have your baby.

The greater the light of your love, the more easily shadows are vanquished forever.

When it comes to family, you're more easily able to set boundaries with [a brother or in-law], or your parents or your husband's parents, for this new chapter of your life it is OK to say no, part of an educational process, which will help establish happiness, love, harmony, peace, enlightenment, boundaries, and proper training, for all individuals involved.

Each and every time you practice this, you perfect it a little bit more, while protecting yourself in even greater and better ways.

All of this becomes an experience of joy, and reeducation of those around you, as needed, whenever needed, mutually beneficial to any and all involved.

Most especially to love yourself now, more truly stress free and enriched, which becomes as an endless for reservoir of love, for yourself, your relationships, your child[ren], and all that is your life.

Any and all of this working out itself more and more, on each and every breath and heartbeat, and each and every time you practice this enjoyably, with greater and better results on your own.

Releasing Fears

Your internal, eternal and adaptive always working in your favor, dynamic effective wise mind, in ways both known and unknown to you, is causing you to change your breathing patterns.

Stress begins to fade to a slow and steady deep soothing rhythm, allowing you to feel centered, peaceful and serene, stress-free.

At the slightest hint of stress, worry, anxiety, panic, fear - this deep and slow steady process instantly begins balancing and restoring you, activating greatest, highest, very best healing and life support.

In this place you are completely free and more than ever before invulnerable to worry, stress, as you now are and forever remain feeling more easily able to take on anything.

You simply begin to trust in life.

For now and forever you are certain that you are in a brand new chapter of your life, re-tuned, reset, recalibrated, doing better and better.

The greater a fear or worry from the past once was, or the greater the disharmony or even upset ever once was, those chapters of your life are now done and finished, as you have moved forever forward, feeling more peaceful and in control, as your body, emotions, mind, and thoughts, have decided to release uncomfortable thoughts, feelings, actions, habits, reactions, anything, that ever once stood in the way of a healthier and better you.

With each and every slow and steady deep breath, with each and every beat of your heart, you have decided to rise up and become mightier than any challenge ever presented to you.

You are now and forever completely able to return back to your vibrant, positive, confident self, re-tuned to a higher focus and potential, achieving the potential, each and every day, more energized with a stable and balanced harmonious energy, while each and every night at bedtime more absolutely able to sleep soundly and restfully, as some deepest recesses inside of you, you now sincerely and truly know that you are more heroic now than ever before.

Perhaps even at times looking forward to the greatest challenges coming your way, as proof to yourself of how mighty you have actually become, for truly, that's who you are, and have always been.

Seizing the moment, you rise up to face opposition, even laughing in the face of adversity as you now recognize and sincerely and truly realize how mighty you have always been.

It is almost as if someone from deep, deep inside of you, has reset a switch, a dial, a thermostat, were computer as some kind, even having opened a valve of some kind to drain off the past and to replenish the future with empowerment and highest greatest potential.

Any time there might be a feeling or a memory of a fear, you'll breath, now so supportive, now so deep and soothing, as flowing life supportive breaths kick in from your belly and ribs, instilling strength, serenity, peace, harmony, life force, the ability to rise up and transcended any moment, cleverly and adaptably with ultimate success.

Iner wisdom is now active and guiding your way, trusting in your life, you feel better than you have in years, almost as if feeling centered as you did in the very best past moments, or even just instead, even better than you did even then.

Your automatic mind working at any and all issues, most especially: Free forever of any and all fear, your trust in life grows by leaps and bounds, almost as if each and every time you go through this exercise on your own, you have done the equivalent of eight, fourteen, nineteen years worth of healing, feeling great inside and out, in ways you will now feel.

Free forever of any and all panic attacks; excessive worry will stop, ending any and all anxiety, depends soothing breathing paves your way to higher and more powerful liberation, freedom and success, keeping serene, calm and peaceful, all things working out and balanced.

Free forever of any and all fear of [XXX], a new rhythm and flow develops from the deepest recesses inside of you working this out on each and every breath and heartbeat, having been re-tuned, reset, and recalibrated, feeling fine.

Free forever of any and all fear of [XXX], now only calm, serene and peaceful, trusting in life once again, and finding clever, an adaptive ways to achieve this.

Releasing anything and everything that needs to be released and let go of in your life regardless of what ever it might be, as those things once stood in the way, you know what is your own way of breaking through here, you are heroic and mighty, and as you have set your mind to this, it is so and remains forever.

Free forever of any and all fear, more easily able put the day and its cares up on a shelf at bedtime, to sleep soundly and restfully.

Free forever of any and all fear of not being able to return back to your vibrant, positive, confident self.

Becoming Calm

The more challenged by the situations in your life that affect you, and most especially by situations challenging those you love, but most especially you, the more your correct response is to simply relax by taking soothing, deep and comfortable relaxation breaths, calming down, creating relaxation while feeling comfortably all over.

And with each and every breath you take, and each and every beat of your heart, your whole body relaxes, your mind relaxes, your muscles relax and even feel like they are melting, even the electrical impulses within those muscles and nerves, discharge comfortably and completely while you relax, as you focus on the fact that tomorrow in fact will be a better day, a better day now at hand, you more comfortable, trusting your life while being more easily able to rise to the top, while remaining calm, comfortably detached, feeling deepest and true, complete and total relief.

You are now more determined than ever to easily and dynamically rise up to face down any challenge, for the mightier the challenge, the even more mightier and heroic you become and remain, comfortable and adaptive, dealing with your life head on, absolutely able to succeed.

A few minutes of deep soothing breath generates complete and total stress relief, better than a one week vacation. Short trips, to comfortable nearby locations, feeling more appropriate and even better, you save money, and completely rejuvenate.

You begin to realize that the challenges of today are things you now more easily face down and rise above, because the mightier heroic part of you is now more capable, and more easily able to rise above any and all challenge, because in the long run little bumps in the road that you are now more easily able to handle, not because they say so, but because in fact it is true.

Anything you once found annoying, you now more readily and easily flow beyond and move forward from.

Your clever and adaptive subconscious mind is now coming up with ideas, methods, and plans, to find gratification and pleasure, reward and fulfillment in ways more constructive and truly beneficial to you, than ever before, the more like giving and sustaining to you while reducing friction even while calm or even while the pressure is high.

You are truly learning and creating ways of reducing pressure and stress while being better to yourself, and in turn, to the people around you love the most.

A better more fulfilled you now emerges, not because I say so, but because it is the nature of your own mind, and therefore it forever is, in ways both known and unknown to you.

You're resolving any and all challenges, almost as if someone from deep, deep inside of you, has reason to switch, the dial, thermostat, or a computer of some kind, allowing you to treat yourself in ways free of self-destruction, in fact truly, treating yourself like someone you love and care about.

The days of self abuse and self punishment are now over. Loving yourself and taking better care of yourself, while you are awake, while you're asleep, even while you are dreaming, now working to your ultimate benefit in magnificent and yet powerfully undiscovered ways.

Your mind relaxes, you trust, your eyes and facial muscles relax, your stomach relaxes you calm down and feel better.

You know this all to be true and more and more real. Healing is taking place and you are feeling fine!

Your clever and adaptive subconscious mind is now coming up with ideas, methods, and plans, to find gratification and pleasure, reward and fulfillment in ways more constructive and truly beneficial to you, than ever before, the more like giving and sustaining to you while reducing friction even while calm or even while the pressure is high.

You are truly learning and creating ways of reducing pressure and stress while being better to yourself, and in turn, to the people around you love the most.

Not because I say so, but because it is the nature of your own mind, and therefore it forever is, in ways both known and unknown to you.

You trust in the very true fact that life, your life is now more beneficially taking care of you and for the greater and mightier the challenge, the greater and grander you are to rise, and eliminate the challenge and become a force of healing and inspirational light, showing inner wisdom and guidance, and so it is and remains, certain and sure, feeling and truly creating and inventing methods of relief, and calming peace.

Life of Peace, Free of Worry

As you relax, float, drift, and dream, truly, you have relaxed your way beyond form of barriers in your life, into a new and better barrier free more enlightened and heroically inspired dynamic, chapter of your life. that which you seek, truly, now becoming yours.

You relax, every thought, every action, each and every idea, now leading step by step, to a better place, as you more easily achieve what you seek, easily including peace and happiness in your life.

You relax, you achieve a deeper and more fulfilling a realization, that your life is an ever more supportive place, not because I say so, but because in fact it is true, as you more easily develop the skills and talents, liberated from deep inside of you, better living and life skills, including living your life free of fear and worry.

Each and every feeling, each and every thought, actively working to improve your life, as you become more and more free, inside and out, in ways more substantial, releasing guilt, and achieving peace, worry free, specifically surrounding the balance and restoration as well as longevity of your health, completely now knowing this to be true in your mind and heart, in every thought, action, reaction, each and every feeling, more and more, this now a new and better part of you, as you are released, forgiven, healed, and learning day by day, night by night, to love yourself even more, even better.

More and more each and every day and night, positive, self-fulfilling, life supporting thoughts dynamically overwhelm any and all now done and finished negative thoughts that had ever occurred in your mind over the years which now forever and always, shall be banished and sent off out into the ether.

Step by step, breath by breath, moment by moment, absolutely, you are easily achieving, dynamically activating, in ways both known and unknown to you, a new acceptance of your life and the world you live in, practically Divinely guided and most definitely in ways unstoppable, adaptive, and creative.

You are feeling a new sense of freedom, truly, you know free, succeeding in learning, failure free, learning or succeeding, problem-free, challenge-oriented, for the greater the challenge, the mightier and bolder, more adaptive and clever, more heroic you truly become.

You now an unstoppable force, as your mind is now and forever set free, and powerfully and absolutely, in ways most effective, in ways both known and unknown to you, completely, as if letting out a deep breath and releasing, while forever forgiving and releasing others, as when you were a child, you now and forever free.

It's almost as if someone from deep, deep inside of you, has permanently, always, and forever, reset, re-tuned, recalibrated you, in ways most important, releasing and balancing as well as creating harmony, restoring balance.

As your inner and outer light vanquishes any darkness, for a new and better, improved you by embracing a higher light, inner and outer, of heart and mind, and a newfound and flowing growing wisdom, which absolutely vanquishes any and all shadows, wherever it may have come from to forever and always release and remove, specific negative thoughts and images.

You now embracing every moment of living and your rejuvenated life, while you now enjoy more and better moments, as you are now, more and more surely have been granted a gift from on high, while restoring health, harmony, balance.

You now free at long last from any and all fears, for the greater the fear, the mightier and more dynamic you become, listening to a greater truth from inside of yourself.

You now the unstoppable one, breaking through, blessing and releasing the past, forgiving any and all of it, just letting it all go, more and more comfortable, feeling relief and release from now finished and done chapters of your life.

Moving onward, feeling better, finding newer and better ways to feel better and better, trusting in your life, trusting in the way you create your life, repelling the negative far, far away and magnetizing the most positive and the possibilities of a more limitless, and inspired existence.

Achieving all that you desire, free at long last of disturbing thoughts, taking better care of yourself, and embracing a masterpiece of a well constructed life, determined to be clever and adaptive at this, in ways known and unknown to you, achieving more easily each and every day, each and every night, breakthroughs.

Certainly, you now more easily able to live your life completely in a knowing embrace of peace and harmony.

Just like a blooming flower in the spring, fresh and new, bright and shiny, so calm and at peace, so relaxed, so one top of the world, this time now yours, this improving, masterpiece of a life of yours, so very supportive, all you do, now and forever.

Free of Skin Picking

You are free of picking on yourself or at yourself. You are fine. You are enough.

You look fine. You are completely enough.

You are treating yourself better and getting only better at taking care of yourself, day by day, night by night, moment by moment, whether with other people or even and most especially if you are alone.

You are in fact becoming free of all repetitive and self-destructive behaviors.

Now relax, deeper and further, further and deeper and in this place of deep, true and profound relaxation, you are now forgiving, both known and unknown events, harsh or negative judgments, criticisms, circumstances and opinions, whether those opinions were yours or someone else's, regardless of where they came from, in order to move into a brighter, healthier, better and more whole chapter of your life.

You are finding newer and better more healthy ways of loving yourself better, releasing past uncomfortable moments, truly doing better than picking on your skin or face.

Free of picking on yourself, feeling fine, upbeat, calm, enough, balanced, loved and wonderful in powerful and effective ways.

You are finding newer and more powerful and effective ways of remaining picking free, gentle, calm, temperate, positive, helpful and productive, free of picking at your face or at any part of yourself, most especially if you are alone or if you might feel a bump on your face or on your neck or another part of your body.

You are free of picking, even if you are or might be feeling obligated to listen to somebody or if you are nervous or angry.

You are in a world that is so busy and so full of people and things, you are now redefining yourself as being surrounded and supported by your life, all of your thoughts, all of your feelings, even the sounds from outside, man-made or from nature, make you realize from deep, deep within that you are supported, you are enough, you are finding newer, better and happier ways to enjoy your life as you open up and make the most of every moment.

Feelings are just feelings, thoughts are just thoughts, and there are times when you can be, hot or cold, tired or energetic, but feelings are just feelings, thoughts are just thoughts, and now yours are being reconditioned to support your every thought, feeling and action in better and more cleaver, powerfully effective and potent, self-supporting ways, finding people, events and circumstances to support you better than ever.

Feeling so upbeat and light-hearted you are becoming a self-assured winner in life.

You are finding new harmonies, a newer and building thriving sense of inner peace, relaxing into greater states of life-support and perfection, calmness, clarity and inner pace, giving yourself a break, loving yourself in better and more profound ways.

Finding better feelings, you remain determined to rise up to meet and beat any and all challenges, feeling a new and ever building sense of joy and optimism, a new and improved sense of accomplishment and optimism, creating a new map of thoughts, feelings and behaviors in your life, a sense of power and joy, sharing only your very best, learning and creating newer ways of liking and loving yourself.

You are now yielding to all of this, learning to love your skin and your appearance, you are enough, you might even in fact feel handsome / pretty, allowing your inner light to shine.

You NEED to take matters into your own hands to feel better about yourself, regardless of event of circumstance, so you do.

It's like when you are in a good mood, feeling on top of the world, the whole world is in your back pocket, tapping into the energy of every past triumph, breakthrough, victory and success you've ever had, imagined or felt.

All of this incredible inspirational energy is upon you right now, allowing you to forever flow into a newer and better chapter of your life, the very best part of your life.

You are meant to be here, vital and important.

This world is a better place because you are here.

You have effectively released a person who glows with positive feelings from within and has a growing and building sense of confidence.

A person who looks attractive regardless of older ways and now embraces newer and more supportive ways that now and forever emerge.

You are in fact, relaxing into such a good way of feeling and living, as wonderful mood rises up to embrace and support you, you are feeling attractive, clever, smart and great to be around, people see you as a friend, just as you see yourself now.

You are your own best friend.

In fact, you are forever healing and doing better and better, moving on, feeling fine.

Overcoming Anxiety and Past Abuse

You are moving into a brand new and better chapter of your life, released, healed, and forgiven, rising above the past, polished, shinier, better, renewed, forgiving completely while completely forgiving, releasing and any all past unpleasant memories, forgiving the past, and any and all past abuse, free of abuse, re-tuned, reset, recalibrated, better than ever, having grown up just a little bit more, perfect, just as needed, free from the past, free at long last, you are and you remain.

The only opinion of you that matters is the one you now lovingly create for yourself.

The opinions of other people, whether negative or destructive, none of your business, and now and forever completely released.

In this brand new and better chapter of your life, you are released, forgiven, stronger, becoming smarter, better, brighter, brilliant, better, whole, better, healed, restored, balanced, relaxed, in fact rejuvenated, and restored.

Your mighty inner hero, the part of you that can pull yourself out of dangerous situations, the part of you that knows how to survive, but now instead however, chooses to live, rises up mightily in your favor to restore you perfectly, in ways complete, known and unknown to you.

For in this place you not only like yourself, but learn to create better ways to love yourself, as all and any adversity, anxiety or worry now flows around and beyond you.

You now, rock steady, like a boulder in the middle of a fast running stream, you have been polished by the experience that is called your life, and you now more determined than ever before, to become and remain better and better.

For when you learn to love yourself better and better, about you, what is there not to like? Liking everything.

You learn to become your own best friend, liking and loving yourself, better than ever before, inventing and creating better ways to take the very best care of yourself, as this now spills over into the world around you.

You repel the negative, and just like a magnet, attracting only the positive and best for yourself, easily able now, more easily able now, to shake yourself off, and rise up mightily, heroic, dynamic, bold, all things that did not serve you in wonderful ways, are now released in favor of things that do support you in the very best of ways.

Truly, those things that did not kill you made you stronger.

You now appreciate the heroic nature of who you are and have always been, and continue to be.

Your life now unfolding and better ways for yourself, in ways best, known and unknown to you.

You begin to trust in the perfection of the way your life unfolds, and learn to love yourself in place of things you once found challenging, you now so much more unlimited, the burden is lifted off, actually feeling a release of energy, and now you are in reality, not because I say so but because in fact it is the nature of your own mind, and therefore it remains true.

Each and every day, each and every night, you're learning to like, love, and appreciate yourself, for within yourself this way you remain, and in this way best you are best taken care of by you.

Your life is your creation, as you relax this moment, you recognize and appreciate the fact that you were meant to be here, you were meant to be here, living in your dreams.

You were meant to do great things, each and every step, each and every breath, each and every heartbeat, to achieve that better and true place.

Whether you realize it or not, you take the ride, rise to the occasion, because you can and do, energetically and faithfully achieving your goals, getting to where you need to be, for the sake of yourself, and those you love most, most especially yourself.

As you relax deeper and further a new thought, truthful thought, a better start, foundational life improving thought, now more your own, in your own way, out of your own way, and the very best of ways.

You are enough, you are meant to be here, you protect yourself, and you reinvent yourself moment by moment to become the best that you can be at your life.

You evolve your life in magnificent ways, being truthful and honest, self loving and appreciated, taking the very best care of yourself.

Your life improves every day, every night, relax, realizing you will get there, you are getting there, perhaps in this moment you are there in future moments adjusting to become even better, this now true so much more now true, easily now you forever.

Your past is officially over, you are free, over, not only having survived it, rather polished by it, fortified, strengthened, your intelligence and self awareness now expanded, self-forgiven, you really are and stay, having learned your lesson, moving on, but now instead even better choose to thrive and succeed.

Each and every person you encounter, you now recognize something there for you to learn from.

You learn to accept life lessons in a more gentle and self appreciative way.

You now taking your life in stride, and in a better place, giving yourself all that you need to break through and survive, live, prosper, and even thrive.

However other people are, you now learn and move on, more easily able to detach from events and circumstances around you, to fortify, you adaptive and strengthened, and love yourself better, regardless of person, event or circumstance.

Your mind now open, you are appreciated and patient, knowing who you are, more and more budding and building self-confidence, liking and loving yourself, now more self esteem and self respect, more enthusiastic about your life, and trusting in the world around you.

More insightful and able to read situations and people around you, releasing imbalance, and more reset and restored.

Your correct response to high stress is to breathe deep, relax your way through it, as newer and better thoughts coalesce within your mind.

You more calm, more patient, having done the equivalent of five to eight years worth of improvement and growth each and every time you repeat this enjoyable exercise and technique on your own, with fluid and adaptive high-impact and noticeable results, working very best and only in your favor, looking forward to it.

Your correct response to any and all stress is to relax, re-energize, rejuvenate, empower your inner hero, learning to like life and appreciating all the learning circumstances in your life all around you at the moment you are now living.

Each and every moment that passes, will never be repeated again, treasuring and relishing your life, more cleverly creating and generating a noticeable balanced emotional state, with a calm, more peaceful stomach.

Breathing soothing relaxation through your naval, each and every day and night, you deep breathe and relax all that is your body, your emotions and mind, into a greater soothing harmony and place of inner and outer strength.

Your mind now open to learn, your emotions now open to enjoy, the small stuff now set aside, as you cleverly create wave of relaxation energy and trust in your life, releasing the smaller stuff.

Long gone are the days of victim-hood, and self-confidence now builds.

You now certainly more self-assured, peaceful, serene, excuse free, taking responsibility for yourself and your life, stubbornly determined to treat yourself and others in better ways.

You now take responsibility for your life, create more calm, peaceful, self-respective and successful life, in better and even best of ways, and create a better masterpiece of an existence, that you were meant to enjoy, as you well meant to be here.

Deep within the recesses of your clever and adaptably highly effective automatic subconscious mind, all of these issues being worked out in your favor, in spite of challenges, because of challenges, you now problem-free and challenge-oriented, failure-free, learning or succeeding, pulling it all together, you just doing better and better.

Stress Management for Tourette Syndrome

So just relax, relax, relax, float and drift and dream.

And as you do, allow your imagination to wander, relax, and while you're relaxed, you flow forward, ever onward, and relax and generate an unstoppable brand new beginning, into a brand new chapter of your life, where all that you are, body, emotions, mind, even spirit, are healing, better and harmonized, in fact, more masterfully under your control than ever before.

As you relax now, simply aRow all that you are, most especially physically, to begin to melt, relax, rest, reset, re-tune and restore.

And as you relax, just a bit deeper and further, as with each and every breath, and each and every heartbeat, you know sense, feel, notice, know, there is an embrace of energy around your body, which seems it feels like golden-white light, surrounding you, embracing you, rejuvenating and restoring you, gently melting into your skin, permeating and penetrating every muscle, every fiber, every molecule and atom of energy that is your body, that becomes your body.

Relaxing and bringing the state of relaxation through every particle of energy, that your body is, or will become, to allow healing and restoration to take place, in the deepest and truest ways possible.

Feel and know, as you sense and embrace this healing energy taking place. Relax, float, drift, dream, feel almost asleep.

In this place, deepest and truest relaxation, your mind relaxes and clears, your breathing calms down, your sinuses clear and drain, your neck and head melts, relaxed, your muscles become comfortable and loose, and limp, like a rag doll.

In this moment your body begins to memorize this feeling of relaxation, as a place to return to, a place to regenerate, a place to calm down, become comfortable, a soothing, healing refuge, and return to, even as quickly as taking several slow and steady breaths on your own.

An image, as if in a movie, as if powerfully in the real world, let your mind and imagination wander to an image, thought, sensation, feeling, or picture of you in a boat.

You are alone in this boat, alone, and you are upon the ocean.

As it sometimes had been with your body, the waves become very agitated and energized.

During all of this, your powerful and unstoppable mind is calm and at peace, as you now realize that in this image, you now firmly know, these waves are under your control, so you decide to calm them down, and they begin to respond, on each and every deep and slow steady breath, and on each and every heartbeat, the golden-white light energy's embrace, all around you, is powerful.

You simply decide to turn down the energy of the waves and make the scene around you tranquil and peaceful.

The water under the boat now becomes like smooth glass.

Your powerful and dynamic, always working in your favor, working any and all of this out, in ways both now and unknown to you, unstoppable and heroically inspired mind, now has the power to turn a turbulent ocean into a serene sheet of glass, so very peaceful, so very calm.

In your mind now, just as it was with the mighty power of the ocean, and with the mightier power of your heroically inspired and unstoppable mind, this powerful mind of yours now turns the muscles in your body into something you can melt just like that or easily control as well.

As your muscles relax, and elongate, on each and every slow and steady breath that you take, as any and all of this becomes more and more not only possible, but more and more easily doable, as you now know this to be unlimited truth and so it is and it remains.

You know, it's almost as if someone from deep, deep inside of you, has permanently and forever reset, re-tuned, or activated in your favor perhaps, a switch, a dial, a thermostat, or a computer of some kind, that instantly restores, releases and relieves stress, completely and deeply, and naturally and actually, in fact and truly, to restore and heal you.

In ways both known and unknown to you, in the most unlimiting and completely effective, unstoppable and insurmountable, high-impact, and breakthrough ways.

As a new dawn for a new day begins in your life, you feel on top of the world, like you have the whole world in your back pocket, winning, or truly just simply doing in getting better and better.

In fact truly, you succeed here, not because I say so, but because it is in fact.

A new day in your life, a moment of true powerful personal healing, the greater energy shifts you away from any and all shadows, as a new harmony of light, both inner and outer is now yours, as you sense, feel, and actually know the embrace of this to be true.

Stress Relief – Stomach Illness Support

It has been said that the mind is the greatest of all healers.

The mind heals the body, the mind reaches beyond time and space, the mind, the human mind, your mind in fact, a place of endless inspiration.

This powerful mind of yours, now relaxes, becomes inspired, and reaches beyond former and now done, no longer permitted unworkable limits, to a place of greater knowing and truth, to a place of higher ability and higher wisdom, higher empowerment and absolute healing, allowing you specifically to tap into higher realms of healing wisdom and inspiration.

All creative abilities generating feelings, now experienced and expressed, enjoying every abundant peace and healing within yourself physically, emotionally, and mentally.

Simply accepting this truth now, knowing this to be true instead, with this higher wisdom and guidance, expressing itself through you and all around you, you now unstoppable, providing only all that you need, while sensing, feeling, and knowing this to be true.

Healing and success, your only options here.

Learning or succeeding, your new pathway to success in this new, uncommonly doing better chapter of your life.

Putting your foot down, digging your heels for obstinate success and breakthrough or, perhaps instead like a wrestling match, having bounced off the ropes, you now rebound, stronger, better, more feisty, unstoppably determined to break through, thrive, and succeed, surmounting all obstacles for the more challenged, the more creative and clever, breaking through you become, with uncommon inspirational brilliance and success.

You relax deeper and further now 3, 2, 1, almost as if someone from deep, deep inside of you, has reset a switch, a dial, a thermostat, or a computer of some kind, only allowing for unlimited and overwhelming health, healing, and beneficial improvement.

As you are now reset, retuned, and recalibrated, you transcend dynamically, above and beyond any upset or anger into everything more beneficial and positive.

That makes you more determined than ever, to rise up, come back, forgive, release, heal, and become heroically mighty, relaxing yet powerful, to allow your appetite to increase while your body remanufactures itself in a healthier and better way.

Perhaps a sense, a feeling, or the embrace, in fact of substantially healing golden-white light, and this light, vanquishes all disharmony and imbalance from your body.

Both large and small, light vanquishes shadows, all over your body, deep within you, and even on a molecular level.

Feel this and sense this warming, healing, soothing, just-right light, on each and every breath and heartbeat, as your appetite now comes back and your stomach, and digestive system and processing, now calm, relaxed, restoring, healing, restoring, healing, and appropriately hungry, more and more life supporting, in better balance, restoring better health inside and out.

Your body, now in a new chapter of your life, of a higher energy and light, shedding the lower energy and imbalances into past chapters of your life, restoring, reenergizing, rebounding, and rebalancing itself.

As you have been reset and retuned, the light within your stomach, spreads down into your intestines and elimination system, drawing more water, lubrication along with any substance that allows you to eliminate imbalance and restore natural rhythm and harmony to eliminate body waste with ease as necessary day or night.

You relax even deeper now as your body seems to melt away as you sink even beneath my words even deeper, not because I say so, but because it simply happens to be.

Pleasantly numbing any area of your body under your control now, yes of course it is, to eliminate any and all discomfort, in ways both known and unknown to you, so very effective, more easily able to succeed while activating comfort within yourself, pleasant numbness, as only your very best, this mighty unstoppable you, is now more than ever before determined to generate light, healing, comfort, into any and all areas you need most.

So very enabled, inspired, thriving, healing and succeeding, filled with light vanquishing and completely removing the shadows, any and all now done and released, forgiven and healed darkness, into places once disturbed, now filled with incredible golden-white light.

Now rebalancing and restoring, healthier and better, now generating in ways both known and unknown to you beneficial, incredible balance and harmony, healing, wholeness and wellness, as you have now discovered within yourself, in ways both known and unknown to you, as it has been said, in fact, that all creatures in the world have the ability to heal themselves, now too so do you.

Your body now more easily generates anything and everything necessary to achieve this, for manufacturing chemicals, redistributing minerals, generating endorphins, applying happy and inspired emotions and thoughts, activating a greater and higher reality around you.

As if breathing golden-white light breaths through your naval, all that is your stomach begins to calm down, become comfortably relax deeper further, more comfortably numb, calm and happy.

Just you feeling better and better, and as a matter of fact, in the back of your mind you knew, you always knew you could, so now activated.

YES you can. And so it is and so it remains.

Relax even deeper this one more time, imagining your body, all that is your body, every part, every limb, every organ, every cell, every molecule, each and every particle of condensed light, now unleashed and more unlimiting, coming to a higher level of energy, truly, activating a higher energy within you, a feeling warming the heart, an inspiration within the mind, fusion of wisdom, expanding this light all around you.

You determined to become lighter, you rising up, simply doing this, you now unstoppable and successful.

Any and all upset, you now process this inspirational energy and dynamic fuel to heal, motivate, restore, generate healing, generating release, forgiveness, any and all discomfort, any and all disharmony, any and all imbalance now released into now former done and finished past chapters of your life.

This new chapter, beginning right now, only becoming brighter, better, more unstoppable each and every day, each and every night, each and every breath, each and every heartbeat, has released the shadows creating light, has released the imbalance restoring harmony, has released the motivational, self-love, eternal peace and harmony, wellness, stress-free and more hyper-motivated you.

Each and every time you sleep, happy pleasant dreams work out these issues for you automatically, as you rest better at night, and in the morning when you awaken, after a deep, and powerful restful and restorative, healthier night's sleep, you are now forgiven and released.

Perfectly inspired and enabled to face down any challenge, for the mightier the challenge, the more heroic and mighty you are motivated and inspired to become, not because I say so, but because it is a fact you have made up your mind to do this.

With every breath, every heartbeat, each and every blink of your eyes, this now so becomes you more.

Each and every little step forward mean a lot, each and every step forward, a new breakthrough for you.

For truly you are released, relaxed, and reidentified, now healthier, brighter, better, capable, forgiven, loved and loving, embraced way inspirational higher wisdom and capabilities, re-energized, of a higher healing light, and so it is, and so it remains, and more easily powerful this becomes for you, better and deeper, each and every time you do this on your own.

Relaxation and Comfort During Pregnancy

As you relax, float, drift, and dream, you're relaxed your way beyond any and all former limits, so comfortably, blockage freed, happily, easily, noticeably, dynamically, into a brand new chapter of your life.

Re-tuned, reset, recalibrated, for any and all uncomfortable actions or reactions are now finished and let go of completely.

You feeling relaxed.

You are free, knowing you are free, you completely transcended any and all uncomfortable past feelings or moments, acting and reacting in better ways, for yourself, and for your child, breaking through here in great measure, breaking through here completely.

You release, you relax, forgive, and let go of anything and everything that had once been in your way, now freed, feeling better, inspired, even great, just healing, forgiving, and releasing, any thought, action, reaction, feeling, than ever once caused you to be overly warm, or maybe just uncomfortable, in any way, in ways both known and unknown to you.

Your body temperature, your skin temperature completely now under your control, after one or two slow and steady deep breaths, imbalanced energy so much more easily released,.

You restored, so much more accurately stabilized, more and more comfortable and calm, your reactions, your feelings, now so much more supportive, so much more inspired, generating effortlessly a balance of body, heart, mind, and emotions.

Sleeping better and more restfully, more successfully, easily, right through the night, more easily able to fall back to sleep, resting deeply, putting the day's cares upon the shelf an hour or two before bedtime, completely unwinding, and relaxing, each and every bedtime.

In this brand new chapter of your life, you more certain, more assured, solid yet adaptive, fluidly generating more supportive feelings, more supportive thoughts, more supportive habits, more supportive desires, more supportive actions, especially reactions, and all that you need to do to take better care of yourself.

Your body so much more comfortable, so much more calm, so much more inspired, so much more enabled, feeling the embrace and support you generate from all around you, of a better life, and better feelings all around you.

In the very best of ways, both known and even unknown to you, you are completely forgiving, healing, released.

It's almost as if someone from deep, deep inside of you has reset a switch, the dial, a thermostat, or released a valve of some kind, easily blowing off any and all imbalance to you, waves of restorative energy now embracing you, just imagining it or maybe just feeling it somehow, ways most important, and of greatest impact, things just getting better and more and more right, generating only more comfortable and ease in all you do.

You are determined to feel better, so simply, you are feeling better.

You now freed and liberated from the past, freed at long last, ahhhhh, you now so completely inspired and empowered.

Any of all of this so much more easily accessible, stable, and under your power, under your control, and any time during the day, but even more so, especially at night, when resting.

You begin to realize that it has been written: Worry is an empty vessel with a hole in it, it does nothing, it holds nothing, it is useless.

Now knowing from deep, deep inside, you now, so worry free now, that each and every thought, each and every feeling, each and every reaction, gears you forward toward inspirations and feelings that only serve you in the very best of ways.

You now feeling stronger and mightier, inspired from every victory, triumph, breakthrough and success you've ever had, your inner hero, the mighty part that is truly capable of great things, the part of you that is capable of saving children from danger, now rises up to the top in the very best of ways, to support you here completely, resolving any and all issues, while you are awake, especially while resting at night peacefully and happily dreaming, restfully and happily sleep, trusting in yourself and your life.

Any thought, any feeling, which no longer serves to empower you, begins to resolve, release, concentrating instead calmly, with steady balanced emotions, with calming, soothing centeredness, rising up, you now mightier than any challenge presented to you in your life from now on.

Now knowing this, this truth, now more your very own, in each and every moment of your life, as so it is, and forever remains, adaptably and fluidly your own now.

Your body chooses to react supportively and in balance, your emotions choose to react, each and every thought, healing, chooses to react, and in truthfully better ways, more supportive, and taking loving care of yourself better, and each and every moment of your life, most especially whatever your condition, most especially whenever pregnant.

You now more trusting in life, you now more fearless, you now more strengthened, you now more supported, externally and internally as well, knowing you are now more brave, courageous, even intrepid, rising up mightily to get the job done here, for having relaxed through former barriers which have now been released into past chapters of your life permanently and forever, you bask by day in the sunshine of a better moment in your life, trusting in the moonlight at night, to rest peacefully knowing a new truth in your life has now emerged, as your body now acts and reacts, in ways that are only self-supporting to you.

Keeping the small stuff small, you focus on tasks at hand taking the very best care of yourself, calm, serene and centered, in ways most meaningful to you, or simply in ways that allow you to a be more effective at any and all of this, getting the job done completely and absolutely.

Your body reacting to your pregnancy in ways only self-supportive, generating the best possible experience for you, as you now can and shall notice truth, in calm self-support, in knowing, glowing confidence, the fact that you have in reality, truly and in fact improved.

You improve, your life improves, your actions, habits and reactions improve, things working out in your favor, you trust in your life and in yourself more, more completely, and better, and each and every way.

And so it is resolved, and so you are, and so it remains forever.

Healing Anger and Creating Calm

You realize that the newer and more correct response to any challenge or stress of any kind is to relax, all that you are, through any and all barriers, choosing responses that generate soothing calmness and healing, most especially whenever challenged by others, choosing in your best interest and in your favor to adapt, rise above, talk it out, resolve, while generating deep and powerful mental and emotional release, relax, focus and take your power back over any situation, trusting in a better outcome, while listening or explaining, generating openness, becoming flexible, adaptive, reducing stress while calmly deep breathing, taking a break, while soothing.

Anger energy responses are fully released by deep breathing, making time to laugh, exercise and in extremely prolonged cases of anger, [writing letters you don't send for release] giving yourself the benefit of the doubt and giving yourself a break, by forgiving yourself.

Inside everyone resides an inner hero, and it's time to redefine yourself that way.

Who you really are is a hero, capable of saving children from great danger like a fire, but beyond past influences, you have allowed yourself to redefine yourself as more than that.

You are now and forever more safe, freed from what you once saw as less than; you now the mighty one in your life, rising up ever onward, to face down the greatest challenges.

From here on out, each and every thought, idea, feeling, concept, each and every plan or action or even reaction, redefines you in the most supportive and self-loving, most unlimited, appreciative of ways.

You now see yourself redefined as released, capable, skillfully maneuvering, victorious, breaking-through, triumphant, successful and empowered, failure free, succeeding and learning.

You are empowered, forgiven and even unstoppable. The power of your breath detaches you dynamically from the moment. You easily achieve a higher place of being and greater piece of mind about yourself and your life.

You are becoming personally more mighty on a daily basis, beyond any and all challenges, while easily rising above old situations and blockages, stress free, relaxed, centered, calm, serene, while powerfully and easily living from newer sense of truth, adaptiveness and inner power.

Self-assured and calm, you are dynamically achieving higher purpose and more balanced states of consciousness, love, true healing, compassion, calmness and limitless joy.

Calmness and serenity now your path, adjusted and achieved by the power always working in your favor, your subconscious mind, in ways both known and unknown to you, in ways most effective, adaptive and correct.

It happens by the power of all you and is easily generated by the energies of what once used to stand in your way, now converted.

Now out of your way, happier, freer and cleverly creative, reset to face all challenges, and so it is and remains, only getting easier and better forever.

You shall get through. You relax, you are one, your emotions begin to settle down, on each and every heartbeat and breath, as your mind quickly clears, calms and centers, or brings you up to the benefits and possibilities of a better moment in a more empowered and inspired you forever arises.

You relax, you unwind, becoming clear and focused, more and more comfortable on each and every heartbeat and breath, as your mind quickly clears to a state of alert calming peace.

You are more inspired and empower than ever before to make this happen, completely adaptive yet stubbornly determined, you break through and mighty in powerful yet deeply fulfilled profound ways.

Your dynamic subconscious mind is working out for you, automatically, but complete ease and effectiveness, treating yourself better, meeting challenges, as you are now treating yourself like someone you love and care about, the days of the torture test in your life now over.

You can easily and cleverly adapt to release feelings of anger or rage and replace them with the experience of calming peace.

It is more important to remain calm and tranquil, clear and focused, to achieve beneficial outcomes and results, as so you do and so it remains.

You give yourself this gift, it remains yours forever. This only becomes stronger, and more beneficial, each and every day and night, while you were awake, while you were asleep, even while you dream, your mind is working this out for you, so inspired, you now unbeatable. For the mightier the challenge, the more clever, and more dynamic, more dear, most heroic you are.

You can easily experience and feel the embrace of the relaxation that you now experience, becoming a permanent part of who you are.

And just after one or two deep and slow steady breaths, your energy shifts and changes, better and profound thoughts and feelings inspire you to break through unbeatably, bringing you right back here, as you need to be here, it now happens to you and it feels wonderful.

You choose to relate to your life and the circumstances around you now connected to your life in a more gentle, loving and self-supporting ways.

You are now believing in yourself, beyond belief, there is faith, beyond faith you are now truly in a new place knowing, a greater and better truth, a more reliable and trusting, inspired and empowered you, is now mightily rising to the top unbeatably here.

Imagine or notice pockets of anger energy, and releasing them as waves of energy from your body, your mind, your emotions, your entire system, in fact, from your entire existence, wave after wave leaving you, draining away, draining away, until you and your life, happier, are more and more free, calm and centered.

What fills these places that once held anger within you, are feelings of life support, optimism, unconditional love, and better feelings, inspirations, upgrades, thoughts, ideas, feelings, that support you, while allowing you to generate a more comfortable, happier, calmer, and centered, more serene and peaceful you.

You notice this, you smile, it's true, you're doing better easily and in ways most meaningful for you. You even notice and appreciate this, you smile, it's good.

Most especially whenever confronted by difficult situations your correct response is to deep breathe, relax, detach slightly from the moment.

You relax, feel inspired, and breakthrough, while remaining calm, peaceful and serene, retaining your focus, and staying centered in your world.

You are in control of your life, and sometimes the best way to control, is to let go, so you do, you detach while remaining completely relaxed and flowing with the situation even releasing and letting go, rather than attempting to control it.

Anger serves no purpose in your life the way it once used to. Right now, you are more determined than ever to remain calm, peaceful and serene, in spite of challenges by things that once made you angry in the past, as you are now certainly in a new chapter of your life, brand new, reset, recalibrated, breaking through.

Any and all tendencies and habits, from past chapters are now done forever from your life. You relax, peaceful and serene, a sea of tranquility. In your mind you now know, from foundational places deepest inside of you, that you are and you remain more calm and focused, finding ways of doing better and better.

You're now focused upon the fact that in this new chapter, things you once considered mistakes, are now and forever learning experiences.

From now on, you only learn, thrive, or succeed, trusting the flow of your life, while remaining calm and centered.

You are inspired, you are empowered, you are completely able, you are relaxed, as your clever adaptive subconscious mind, is now reset, recalibrated, rejuvenated, relaxed, releasing, and letting go.

You now feeling fine, doing better, all of this getting better and better. Whether the news is good or bad, you relax, you are cleverly inspired, you are breaking through, and your mind and emotions, here right now breaks through unbeatably.

For the greater the challenge, the mightier are, you now are and become forever. You begin to rely upon and trust within yourself and your life, and the way your life now unfolds.

The mighty inner hero, the part that's capable of saving children from great danger, like a fire, easily now steps forward, and all of the greatest challenges you have ever faced, see yourself and the mighty hero that you are.

Any time you're in front of a large group, you know these people are secretly cheering you on, secretly fans, wishing for you to succeed, so now you relax, feel at home, you deep breathe, and so you do.

Whether with your people or alone, your life allows you to thrive in ways yet unimagined, relaxing through barriers now, you're more challenge free, barrier free, flowing in mightier than ever before.

Where you used to scream, you now choose deep breathing, slow and steady breaths, to release emotion calmly, grow up more peacefully, and transcend any and all limits, becoming a mighty leader, calm, cool, focused, direct, explaining, reasoning, loving yourself enough to succeed, and working like a leader to direct others, explaining it better, free of frictional games, free of ever struggling or trying.

Simply do what is right and avoid what is wrong, while developing Saint-like patience, allowing yourself to relax into a brand new chapter of your life, uplifted, for the stronger the adversity, the more mighty, dynamic, peaceful and powerful you are, a shining example to everyone who knows you.

Insomnia – Better Sleep – Better Rest

When it's time for sleep, and it's time for bed, it's time for sleep, time for rest.

Time to put the day up on the shelf, time to relax, rejuvenate, and feel a blanket of soothing, healing, relaxation energy, embrace you as your whole body slumps down, into an unwinding, soothing, healing, relaxation state, as the day's cares and challenges are put up on a shelf an hour or two before bedtime as the day is done, and you strictly allow yourself to relax and become rejuvenated by a blissful night and a deepening, rest and sleep.

Just as you have done so many times in the past, you simply put your head down upon the pillow, close your eyes, and sleep, activating the well-remembered, sweet embrace of sleep; now so much more easily.

Ever more easily gotten too, and the more easily effective.

You relax and your dreams become carefully crafted and adaptive toward working out any issues, all issues, in your favor, as you rest deeply, easily, peacefully, and naturally, well-deserved, more trusting in your life.

As it's time for bed, any and all challenges, in fact the greater and mightier the challenge, the more your body unwinds, to compensate and generate well deserved rest, from now on, as a new, more heroic, more inspired, more capable, more motivated, more easily able to rise up, chapter of your life has now begun; you now the unbeatable one.

For whatever the challenge has been during the day, for the greater the challenge, the mightier you become and the more easily able you are to manifest improvement, in both ways known and unknown to you.

As your mind clears and becomes super-relaxed, as any and all challenges, even symptoms begin to become pleasantly released, become pleasantly numb and under your control to truly allow you better and complete rest, as the various aspects of your body begin to become pleasantly numb and unwind, unwinding and unwound, as any and all outside influences seem to be fading away, you become even better, even great, and relaxing your way beyond any and all challenges.

Sleep, sleep at long last.

Always free of over-thinking at bedtime, you recognize it is your duty, right, so well deserved, to get an important and powerful, peaceful night of rest, to be at your very best tomorrow and all tomorrow's, at your best both any day or night.

As the sleep, your restful wonderful sleep, deep and heavy, so well deserved that you now truthfully and truly feel this completely upon you at this place in this moment, easily now memorized as a place to return to, coming upon you more easily, as you relax, rest, float, and dream, doing better and better each and every day and night.

No real place to get to, just a place of peace and rest you now can generate on your own.

Your mind now clears, your body unwinds, you set up and develop rhythms, pathways, step by step methods and processes, to allow all of you a deeper, calmer, more rejuvenating, more wonderful time to rest.

And each and every time that you repeat this enjoyable exercise, as a pathway back to a deeper more rejuvenated you, it becomes quicker, deeper, easier, more effective, with greater impact, each and every time you do this on your own.

Your always clever and dynamic adaptive mind, is now working out beneficial ideas, methods, pathways, solutions, adaptations and improvements, to generate success in these ways.

Most effectively and easily, generating complete and ultimate success, in ways both known and unknown to you, and so it is, and so it remains, and therefore you succeed.

Claustrophobia Extra

You have risen up and decided to become mighty, in the face of any and all challenge, even adversity, choosing to feel comfortable, peaceful and serene, almost as if someone from deep, deep inside of you, as reset a switch, a thermostat, or dial of some kind, even a computer, which allows you to become and forever remain, peaceful, calm, most especially when ever entering any kind of a tunnel, an elevator, a small public bathroom, choosing to relax and feel your energy shift into a place of deep profound serenity.

Learning Enhancements

College Concentration, Memorization, Memory and Leadership

As you relax, and float, drift and dream, while feeling deeply and truly relaxed, a true sense of inspirational and soothing calmness is upon you, as an absolutely wonderful new thought begins to arise in your mind, a knowing and glowing thought, that truly, you have entered a brand new chapter of your life, feeling mightier and more adaptive, more easily able to rise above and fully and forever transcend, all of the things that ever once stood in your way.

In this new chapter of your life, you have made and continue to make, deep and profound adjustments and improvements, recognizing these improvements, and making them your very own. Your correct response to any and all situations that once ever caused you any kind of stress, is to relax, taking deep and slow, steady breaths, as you feel, sense and truly now are able to generate when necessary and only know the embrace of, a more stress-free, and relaxed you.

As you begin to breathe slowly and deeply, there is a shift in the energy within your body, feeling and knowing this improvement, to step forward boldly and to achieve all desired outcomes. Most especially, maintaining interest and excitement are profound breakthrough life goals, of achieving and excellent grades in college and acquiring the well-deserved reward of a college degree.

You begin to concentrate on your schoolwork, because as you relax to beyond all barriers into a brand new chapter of your life, you have adjusted your thinking, and are now whether you realize it or not, finding things to become and remain forever interested and even fascinated about.

Perhaps it is the material, perhaps it is the facts, perhaps it is skillfully understanding how the system you of being taught works. Perhaps it is understanding the lay of the land in that system, maybe it's even the way the professor is explaining the material, or maybe even it's just like someone from deep, deep inside of you , has reset the switch, the dial, the thermostat, a computer of some kind.

Which in this brand new, recalibrated, reset, and improved chapter of your life, your mind has now become like a sponge, absorbing any and all information, or perhaps more like a computer, working in your favor, adaptively and cleverly easily able to achieve, create and generate memory, comprehension and recall, while relaxing beyond former limits, excited about new ideas and concepts, easily able to adaptively and cleverly retrieve information, while easily being able to reason new understandings and points of view, that allow you optimal outcomes, breakthroughs and successes here.

Even as you sleep at night, you rest peacefully, trusting in the fact that your now reconditioned mind, even better functioning thought processes, and even more self-supporting emotional reactions that are now working in your favor to break you unbeatably and mightily through here, allowing even restful peaceful night's sleep, as even your pleasant dreams, peacefully, allow you to cleverly and skillfully melt away and easily flow beyond, any and all old barriers, both known and unknown to you that now seem to be dissolving and melting away.

As your ability to concentrate, reason and to cleverly adapt, feel inspired and succeed, remember, perform, recall, maintain high levels of interest, are all now coming together in appropriate measured response, to break you through here unbeatably and successfully, generating and creating the kind of breakthrough success, you truly deserve, as you have now unstoppably decided and determined, that this is a gift of success and triumphant victory you have now chosen and to give yourself.

As you relax and embrace this new chapter of your life, your ability to concentrate and focus seems to be with laser like precision. You attend the classes, you read and perform and remember and concentrate and most especially retrieve and recall effectively and as needed, while making success your own. For what used to be, you are now better at. For what used to be, you are doing better than.

You relax and allow your mind now to work in your favor, not because I say so, but it is because you have made a decision and in fact truly, it is the nature of your own mind to do this. Your memory now sharp and clear, trusting in the fact that you are only able to remember, perform, recall, not only from whatever you've read, as well as what you've heard in the lectures, while remembering dates and events and whatever else may be needed at any time.

You are even easily allowing yourself to trust in memories that spark to mind as needed whenever an answer is needed. You are becoming one with the idea that it is time to succeed, and you've given yourself this as a gift, not only just for yourself, but for those you love, and those who love you, but most especially for yourself. It feels great to get out of your own way and to simply thrive and succeed here.

You allow your mind to work in fully functional ways, including photographically, to recall, retain, retrain, as well as retrieve, any image, any thought, any concept, and the powerful feeling, that allows you more interest, that a memory, and limitless scholastic success.

From deep inside of you, the parts of you that are both doubtless and dynamic, rises to the very top, to lead your way to success. Whether it's school or work, you are available to draw up from deep, deep inside of you and liberating out into the world around you, your ability to lead, direct, and manage, courageously trusting in your ability to focus, sense, feel, know, how to delegate, arrange, and become a team leader and organizer, by encouraging and relaxing beyond any and all in balance, into a comfortable yet motivated and skillful leader, who expresses, guides, explains, educates, expresses insights, is a good listener and adaptive personality type, who inspires others, and motivates others to fulfill the greatest potentials. All of this happening around you as if it's second nature to you.

Test Taking, Recall, Retention, Passing

As you are studying for your test, your correct response to any and all challenges is to react way beyond those challenges into a brand new chapter of your life which surprisingly and amazingly has begun right now in this moment, only getting more effective and stronger, beyond all doubt, undoubtedly sure and certain and assured that a brand new chapter of your life has unbeatably begun right now where things that once stood in your way are now in the past, as you are blockage free, calm and focused, ready to move forward and seize your moment of success, right here and now.

Your powerful, adaptive, always working in your favor mind, right now, powerfully has been reset, recalibrated, retuned, refocused, almost as if someone from deep, deep inside of you has reset a switch, a dial, or a thermostat of some kind that is now and forever unlimiting you, unleashing your mighty inner hero, the part of you that knows no doubt nor fear, to bring you right here unbeatably into a better place in your life now.

Retaining all that you have ever heard, read or experienced, or imagined, whenever you need it, to bring right here unbeatably into a better place in your life now, only retaining, recalling, and performing with the skill of the master, the ability to retain all of the information that you are reading.

Not because I say so, because it is the nature of your own of new and improved dynamic mind to do this, all of this working in your favor, while you are awake, while you were asleep, and even while you were pleasantly and supportively dreaming, your mind is inventing success strategies both known and unknown to you, and you trust in the fact this is happening for you, almost as if it is happening all around you, inspired and unbeatably and it feels wonderful.

For in this moment this is your truth. Your mind now responding like a powerful computer, with attention, sharp focus, and an unbeatable ability to break through here, remembering, recalling, performing, and even trusting in your first instinct and impression of an answer to any question, while free of over-analyzing, while at the same time having an understanding of a lay of the land, which is to say, understanding the system, well enough to be able to even reason out answers, as you are now confidently understanding the rhythm and the pace of the subject matter at hand, feeling wonderful. All of this getting easier and better for you dynamically, feeling driven forward to succeed.

In your mind now, imagine what a successful you looks like. How you feel, how you move, how you walk, how you sit, how you work, how you relax, feel confident, how you get through the day, and how feeling so deeply strong, and confident, you drift off at night into a deep restful sleep, embraced by relaxation, in body, emotions, mind, and even spirit, powerful and embracing soothing harmony, dreaming wonderful happy and supportive dreams, awakening at a proper time of the morning, ready to seize the day and happy about life.

Make this sense and image stronger and stronger as you allow it to become one with you, this future you, who has broken through here, inspired and succeeding dramatically, all things working in success harmony, having done the work, broken through skillfully and with confident, glowing, complete success, and has responded like a professional, for truly, what the pros know you know, what they do, you do, how they react, you react, how they are inspired, you are inspired, how they succeed, you succeed, how they break through, you break through, almost as if this has already happened.

You you deserve this, and you make it your own, because now, you realize that you are mightier than any challenge ever presented to you in your life, and when compared to some past challenges of your life, when against the odds, you confidently rose above, vanquished or embraced, and succeeded completely, in spite of or because of the conflict, with the appropriate warm, confident energy all around you at that moment, which is around you now, feeling its embrace.

You now, thriving, memory, recall, performance, drive, determination, strength, reasoning, focus, in the zone, in the moment, getting only stronger and better, on each and every breath and heart-beat, breaking through here unbeatably, heroically, unstoppably, while you are completely now and forever glowing in life-force harmony, the harmony of heart and mind, because you have decided to make all of this your own and so now it is, a fact, a truth, your reality, doing all that it honestly takes to step forward and make success your very own.

In fact, youre correct response to any and all stress, is to deep breathe soothing breaths, and feel an upward shift in your energy, the energy of your heart and mind, like an energy ball around your body, the energy of all that is in the room with you, people, objects, even the air around you seems charged with the energy of inspirational success, while you are feeling so confident and serene, so very able, more and more than ever before, because you are, and whether you get realize it or not, you have become completely unbeatable.

In your mind, in your heart, in all that you are physically, mentally, emotionally, even spiritually, a harmony that allows you to transcend any and all limitations, now rendering you limitless, is now breaking you through right here and right now, as you now look forward to taking on any and all challenges, for the greater the challenge, the more mighty, dynamic, centered, serene, guided, unstoppably striving forward and ultimately successful and inspired you are, rising to the very top, taking on all things and taking things in stride.

Of course you are and now you do, and achieving a passing grade or even just simply unbeatable success, while taking this on and making it your own, completely overwhelming any challenge. You are now the mighty one, an unstoppable force, and it feels so good.

Each and very time you repeat this wonderful technique on your own, all of this is getting more flexible, and adaptive, effective and successful, more inspired and driven, powerful, focused, and unbeatable, not because I say so, but because it is the nature of your own dynamic mind to do so, for you have succeeded, you are living in a place of unbeatable, inspired power, and so now and forever it is and remains yours.

Better Test Taking - 1

Your mind easily becomes reoriented, almost as if someone from deep, deep inside of you has reset a switch, a dial, a thermostat, or a computer of some kind, and now you easily have better memory and recall, free from any and all effort, it simply happens.

You relax, calming mind and body, emotions, mind and spirit, as all of you resets itself to a greater level of calmness and ease, almost like you'd been doing this for 10, 20, 30 years, except now knowing the more limitless power is within you,.

Any and all of this take you to a new to and better place, as every thought, feeling, and emotion, realigns itself to support you and break you through as a successful test taker.

Almost like being divinely guided, almost like being guided from on high, all of this begins to happen around you unbeatably.

All that is your long- and short-term memory steps forth, while you are beginning to trust in your first answer, first impulse, first choice, free of over-analyzing, relaxing as the answers become easier, is correct and precisely focused.

Your mind, now refocused and precise, easily remembering, recalling, answering and performing precisely, everything you've ever read, heard, studied, solved, trusting instinctively in your answers.

Giving yourself this precious gift, you remain free of procrastination or anxiety, finishing whatever you start, motivated to succeed, ready to rise up and be mighty, rising up to the top of the hill, coasting your way down, getting the job done, heroically, not because I say so, but because it is the nature of things, you, and your own mind to do this, and so it is and so remains.

Knowing the new integrated truth in your life, as budding and building self confidence triggers a success inspired, failure-free, worry-free you, so calm and peaceful, so in the zone of testing success.

Feeling this and knowing this, now is the time, success is yours, as you feel the energy of success all around you, as you now more easily than ever before, take each test with confidence, answer each question instinctively, sailing through calmly and with assurance, going the whole nine yards with unstoppable inspiration, a sense of mastery, mightier than any and all challenges you might face, looking forward to facing them down, feeling serene, unbeatable, and free.

Any and all of this is now yours forever, and so it is and so remains, liberating a future you, who was already succeeded.

Doing only all of your very best, especially for yourself, even more especially for those people you love, but even more especially for yourself, having broken through here, your only choice now success, as memory, performance, recall, is yours now.

It's almost like, what the people who wrote the test know, you now know, what they do, you do, how they are, you are, how they are inspired, so too are you.

Your automatic mind, rehearsing this and working out and any and all issues, completely and in your ultimate favor, at all moments, awake, asleep, and even while dreaming, in unstoppable success, in ways both known and unknown to you and it's easy now, and you now know this.

You go forward with the wisdom of your years as well as the clarity and scholastic ambition of a younger [man, woman], your mind so full of knowledge, so clear and sharp, so very focused, so motivated to success, thriving.

Excited and looking forward to your success, you seize the moment, take on the challenge, relaxed, breaking through, succeeding, this is yours now, more certain and more sure than ever before in your life.

The dynamic power of your automatic mind, working this out while you're asleep, while you're awake, even what you dream, every breath and heartbeat lead you to ultimate breakthrough in success here now, feeling heroic and mighty and unbeatable.

Better Test-Taking - 2

As you relax your mind is now wide open to possibilities of only success. Relax and flow and remember, and truly know, ever deeper realizing that all information, any information, and along with the ability you mightily have to reason to something, is currently stored within your mind effectively, easily retrievable, and completely usable, trusting your first impression to anything you might encounter.

For the mightier the challenge, the greater your passion to succeed, in precise and focused ways.

For what any and all of those who have gone before you know, you know, for what they needed to accomplished to pass, so now you do too.

For in some future moment, you have already passed, with a wonderful score. In your imagination, see this future you, glowing with success, admiring yourself while having achieved the respect and admiration of others, glowing in both heart and mind.

In your imagination, float forward now, and step forward and merge into you that you are now, as well as into this now future you, and seize the moment, your future moment, your success, well-deserved and now created.

For in this moment, if you are upbeat, you are unbelievably effective, succeeding and thriving, in a brand new chapter of your life, where success is only the very best option, and the only choice you make.

It is almost as if someone from deep, deep inside of you, has reset a switch, a dial, a thermostat, or a computer of some kind of valve, activating only glowing and flowing assured success, every thought, every feeling, every action, every reaction, every movement of your body, every thought, focused or even wandering, generates only optimum success.

All issues that once blocked or once stood in the way, are now and certainly forever surely, shunted into a past chapter of your life, and now done.

And as it was with you as a child, things from the past, now in the past, now done, while you are free, upbeat, happily looking forward to the challenge so you win, and skillfully and succeeding optimally.

Knowing this you become an unstoppable force of success, knowing this from places deepest within you, right down to your bones, your energy, has up shifted, to a higher register, a place where you now and forever unbeatably succeed.

All things are in the correct measure, studying just the right amount of time, trusting your first instinct and impression as the correct one. Free of over-thinking, you shun the past and smile forward into success both inside and out.

The past now done, passing this test is not only a choice, but a passionate truth that you now live from.

Each and every breath whole and healing, balancing emotion, inner peace and wholeness, a glowing knowing, generating success, letting go of old frustrations, now a part of that past chapter. Now you are finished, you're moving forward, you are liberated, safe, strong, and succeeding here unbeatably.

Like a mighty and unstoppable hero from ancient times, you're motivated and embraced by the energy of every past victory, triumph, breakthrough, and thrivingly unbeatable success, you ever had, or anyone who has ever taken this test has ever had, it is now yours, and on each and every breath, each and every heartbeat, every movement of your fingers, and every naturally occurring blink of your eyes, every day and every night, while you are awake, while you were asleep, even while you dream, peaceful happy dreams, any and all things, generating success here.

You are more certain of this and becoming more and more certain of this than ever before, than any other thing that has ever happened in your life. Not because I say so, but because it is the nature of your own mind to do this, and so this is and it remains as the truth to you.

A new sense of life and thriving is now yours. You have done the work, the information and success, the knowledge and knowing, the intelligence, all of it takes to do this, from places both known and unknown to you, from deep truthful places with a new, and in higher parts of the universe, are all embracing you, driving you forward to break through success, imprecise fashion and skill, knowledge and wisdom, and more certain and sure of yourself, than ever before.

Retaining information, your mind is like a steel trap. All things in balance, you have studied and studied well and the information is there, easily utilized and retrievable as needed, while you are able to recall the answers at will.

Now knowing a higher truth, passing this as anything you put your mind to as a test, now more easily than ever before within your grasp.

Heroically freed, you now venture ever onward to seize your success and make it one with you, making success yours, while enjoying feelings of satisfaction and success, as a deep and true part of you now knows this and makes this all your very own. Having done all of the necessary work, succeeding brilliantly.

Test Taking – Your Moment of Power - 3

Almost as if moving forward in time seven to eight years, almost like having studied an additional seven to eight years, your focus becomes laser-beam precise, as you now more than ever before, easily navigate any test, free of distractions from past events and issues now done, as if they too are seven to eight years back and forever done, and as a result both mentally, emotionally, in ways most effective and important.

Just like the things of your childhood, which seemed important to you then, so much less important to you now, just like letting go of a deep breath, all things once distracting and anxiety provoking, are now done and finished, let go of, healed, and resolved.

While you let go, you absolutely and completely relax, your mind now more clear and more open, more precise and effective, more motivated to rise above any and all challenges, problem-free, distraction free, moving forward, unbeatable, heroically inspired, redefined and more unlimited, all things working in your favor, you now, more certain, more serene, more singularly focused, more easily able to achieve, than ever before in your life.

Now as an adult, you choose to study earnestly and energetically, while taking better care of yourself, preparing yourself and your life, with the pacing, leadership, discipline, that a highly motivated and effective adult uses to accelerate, fine tune, and take the best care of yourself, while being upbeat, able, performing, actively sizing opportunities, and looking forward to taking on any and all challenges.

Loving yourself even more, taking better care of yourself, giving yourself what you now deserve, and make your own, you establish patterns, habits, actions and reactions, that allow you the skill and better best habits, including study habits, smiling to your own benefit and breakthrough.

Within the recesses of your mind, a vast storehouse of knowledge, for everything you have read, everything you have heard, everything you have even imagined, is stored there, more easily accessed now, and activated, most especially whenever needed, by your ability to realize that you are in fact, heroic.

So easily able to trust in your instincts, your first impression generally the correct one and choice, activating memory, precise performance, and while the easily achieving breakthrough, beneficial outcomes, easily retrieving any and all information and inspiration, through slow and steady soothing, stress-free, deep breath patterns.

All of this and any of this, not because I say so, but because it is happening to you all around you, most serenely, certainly, and assuredly, because you have made important life improving decision to move forward, more certain than ever before.

Releasing and shattering past blockages, now and forever freed, and taking and making, living in a brand new chapter of success, beneficially excited, while raising up to meet any and all challenges.

All the information is there, your breath is soothing and calming, you relax, what you need comes back.

In this brand new and more exciting, success motivated, breakthrough chapter of your life, you treat yourself with greater and greater self respect, as your belief in yourself as well as self-esteem rises, and your ability to excel and rise above all, as you right here and now, absolutely know, really and truly know now, you are actually looking forward to taking on and resolving all and any challenges, problem-free, blossoming forth, from places deepest inside of you.

You now know this and live from this moment, your moment of power.

It feels so great to be out of your own way; and so it is, and so it remains now and forever.

Doing anything and everything that it takes to honestly rise up and succeed.

Right choices are made, correct first impressions are followed, while your ability to reason out challenges, correctly rising up and focusing, breaking through successfully, in ways that are most effective, correct, precise, and working in your favor now effortlessly flow forward.

You trust in the fact and in yourself, that life is improving, your mind and emotions now work in your favor as your life now becomes better and better, feeling so good to be free at long last.

Any and all of this getting better and better, each and every time you repeat this wonderfully enjoyable relaxation technique on your own.

Bar Exam Success

As you relax, thrive and succeed, relaxing even deeper, your imagination opens up, activating your mighty inner hero, the part of you that is doubtless, fearless, focused, and completely inspired while enabled, to break you through here.

The greater the challenge, your correct response is to relax, and allow your mind to become completely open. Your always effective, dynamic and wise mind, is now able to overcome any challenge presented to you, most especially the bar exam.

So relaxed, so open minded, so inspired, performing like a pro.

For what the pros know, you know, what they do, you do, how they are able, you are enabled, how they succeed and breakthrough, you succeed and breakthrough.

Slow and steady breath calms, soothes, and restores you, regular heartbeats dynamically guide your way to ultimate success, beyond even what these words mean, to a place of feeling, even knowing.

You now know any and all of this to be adaptably clever and true for you always.

You have done all the learning, you have done all the studying, your mind now stores and more easily retrieves any and all information.

As you deep breathe and relax, your mind opens up, your imagination remains clear and sharp, focused, inspired, able, liberating a future moment of a successful you into the right here and now, the you that has already passed and succeeded.

It's almost as if someone from deep, deep inside of you has reset a switch, a dial, a thermostat of some kind, even a computer into activation, reactivating your enthusiasm as well as your drive and motivation to study.

Your mind so much sharper, so much clearer, so much more driven, enabled, and more easily able to *focus, focus, focus,* laser-beam like precise, easily able to remember, perform, recall, even understand the landscape, to reason out any and all answers as necessary and as needed, while you have memorized and now know, trusting in your first answer and response as the correct one almost always.

You now and forever, free of second guessing and over-reading.

Re-infused, re-enthusiastic and re-excited, approaching that point to ultimate success and the achievement of heroic, breakthrough conclusion.

You now the unstoppable force, truly. You achieve all outcomes as a gift to yourself, loving yourself enough to give yourself these gifts and relishing the breakthrough success you now enjoy and create.

Forever and always now a brand new and better chapter of your life, you take even better care of yourself, motivated to succeed, to recall, read, absorb, remember, perform with optimal precision, even exercise your body and mind, enjoying beneficial energy, and limitless benefit in other ways, as your mind now clear, sharp, focused, allows you to breakthrough here unbeatably.

Any and all of this allows you and even drives you forward to this giving you the energy you need to get up and study.

Better Driving and Concentration for New Drivers

As you relax and float, and drift and dream, you're finding and creating more clever and adaptive ways to be interested in what you are focusing upon, focusing in and upon any and all aspects for safe and proper driving while maintaining safety, whenever operating a motor vehicle of any kind.

Your mind and concentration relax, you maintain proper focus, you are calm, get focused, peaceful yet serene, easily concentrating, focusing, while tuning out any and all distractions, relaxing and maintaining proper distance and safety, as well as optimum skills while driving.

It's almost as if someone from deep, deep inside of you, has reset a switch, a dial, a thermostat, or a computer of some kind, that allows for clarity, focus, awareness of surroundings, while maintaining a proper safety zone around yourself, and your vehicle, free of any and all distractions, laser-beam like precise, maintaining safe distance and agility, focus, flow, rhythm, and concentration, while operating a car or any sort of a motor vehicle.

You have done the learning, you activate highest awareness and skill while remaining relaxed, and in calmness, a peaceful state of relaxed and focused concentration.

Your very best coming up to the surface now, all within your grasp, all within your ability and power to break you through here, and so it is and remains.

You maintain safety and distance from other drivers, and of road conditions, observing and recognizing the signs, and signals of the road, carefully obeying the rules of the road, liberating from deepest places inside yourself, the very best driver you can be.

Activating skill and talent, while maintaining good and proper judgment, and safety distance, free of tailgating, free of dangerous moves, maintaining safety and space, always signaling, breaking at the proper time, being cautious, checking distance from other cars, most especially while turning into oncoming traffic, signaling carefully while switching lanes, navigating carefully, observing and even quickly adapting to changing circumstances, combinations of vehicles, weather conditions, road conditions, doing everything it takes to persevere in becoming and liberating from deepest places inside the best driver you can be.

It's almost as if you've relaxed into a greater state of concentration releasing distraction and childishness, activating greater levels of adult focus and awareness, almost professionally, simply doing and becoming better and better.

Free of cockiness, you have stepped up, become stronger, clearer, you stay calm and relaxed and focused, more easily able to skillfully succeeded this, ever more determined to maintain safety, and awareness, trusting in your actions and reactions, as if they too were re-tuned, while easily and more correctly, skillfully and dynamically anticipating what other drivers might do.

Appreciating and understanding it's more important to avoid an accident than to be right while driving.

It's almost like driving at the proper speeds and in the proper way makes you feel better about who you are inside, so therefore you simply do it and it is.

Your mind relaxes, focuses, opens up, you're more easily able to interpret signs, and directions, while anticipating correctly all around you, adjusting to and getting ready for any lane change that may be coming up, staying calm and choosing safety first.

Remaining free of nervousness and staying calm most especially whenever challenged under pressure from other inpatient drivers.

What other drivers emotions are is none of your business, you're more and only focused and concerned with safety and sanity while driving, and maintaining your health and safety, with a generous love you have for yourself and for your passengers, taking better care of yourself and the people you love most.

Being aware of the poor reactions of other people, even the savage nature of those around you, while you stay in the zone of safety, serenity, calmness, and peace, skillfully and carefully maintaining speed, safety, distance, judgment, always signaling, breaking at the proper times, adjusting to any and all conditions, whether they be traffic, other drivers, hazards in the road, weather, day or night, changes in conditions both expected and unexpected, everything and anything.

Your mind now cleverly and clearly seeks out and relaxes into any and all of this in the very best and most effective of ways, you now open and skillful, re-identified and actually doing better and better, more and more determined, barrier free, because you are now more concerned with safety and better than ever before in your life, and so therefore it more easily is forever remains.

You realize the car is not a toy, driving is a serious thing, an adult responsibility you rise up to meet and succeed at, paying attention as if your life depended upon it, as it surely does.

You take the very best care of yourself, doing everything and anything that it takes to honestly breakthrough here and succeed, and therefore it is and it therefore there remains in your favor.

You remain, and stay serene while carefully driving, more self-observant, even self-assured, as you release nervousness and maintain focus.

Any and all of this is working out better and better in your dynamic, automatic mind while you are awake, while you are relaxing, even while asleep and having happy and peaceful dreams, your mind and all of your consciousness, thoughts, feelings, actions, emotions and reactions, are all working out in your favor to optimum benefit in unlimited ways, for all those who are concerned with you.

Whenever driving, you are always remaining free of getting even, free of road rage, as you are and as you cleverly remain determined to become the best driver you can be.

There is always room for improvement, you decide to improve yourself each and every time you drive, getting better and better, more skillful, more and more of a safe, sane and defensive driver.

You reset, re-tune, recalibrate, for optimum performance, any and all of your concentration, in ways both known and unknown to you as yet, now forever more and more focused and more crystal clear, your judgment becomes better and better, free of second guessing, free flowing while driving, you are more confident, and almost like each and every time you repeat this wonderful exercise and technique on your own, you enhance your experience by several years.

Each and every time you drive you learn something and choose to do better next time.

Showing yourself and the world better judgment, you take better care of yourself and for all concerned, you listen and interpret any and all information, as a part of self improvement while improving your driving skills and tactics, techniques and methods,.

Better and better each and every time you get behind the wheel or if you are even a passenger in someone else's car or in any kind of a vehicle.

You care, you take better care of yourself, your mind is open, sharp, focused and clear, you are self-aware, aware of others, understanding better and better.

You have set your mind to this, and you are doing better and better.

For the greater challenge and circumstance, the mightier and more determined, the more heroically inspired you are,to breakthrough here.

Seizing the unstoppable inspiration in this moment and empowering yourself, you release barriers from the past and flow ever onward, ever more certain and self-assured knowing all of this to be true.

Becoming a Better Reader

As you relax and float, and drift and dream, you're finding and creating more clever and adaptive ways to be interested in what you are focusing upon, more interested in every aspect in detail, almost like it's a game, or something of great interest to you, even if it's work related, as you are now finding yourself to be more excited about picking up and reading a book.

You have now moved into a brand new better chapter of your life, the new thoughts, feelings, and ideas, allow you to shake off the blockages of the now done and forever over past, while releasing boredom, and finding excitement and interest, your mind now more carefully re-tuned and refocused, than ever before, not because I say so, but because it is nature of your own mind to do this, and therefore it is and it remains.

In this new and improved chapter of your life, you are now becoming more aware of your control, and it becomes easier for you to adapt to and deal with things, like reading, and not get bored halfway though it.

You, now reset, retuned and, and recalibrated, more easily able to focus on anything that you put your mind to, knowing that what you are putting your mind you, is in your best interest.

Aaahh, it feel so great to be so free. It is almost like someone from deep, deep inside of you has reset a switch, the dial, were thermostat of some kind, as you achieve all desired results and outcomes more easily, achieving anything and everything that you want, and all that you need.

You are now so easily able to focus and concentrate on a book and retain all it's information. Almost like anything that you pick up is of great interest to you, and your eyes drinking information, as you experience in some way that is extremely interesting and comfortable to you, benefit you mentally, emotionally, in fact, comfortably, in every way.

It is almost as if you have done the emotional equivalent of growing up and achieving a greater level of inner peace, laser-beam like focus, the ability to achieve all that you set your mind to, even wisdom, interest and focus, to the tune of sixteen, seventeen, even eighteen years worth of greater ability, and interest, even discipline, when it comes to reading and even more completely able and capable of finishing a book, before the deadline.

You ignore anything and everything that once stood in your way, now employing the discipline to set the pace, achieve your place, and get the job done.

You now being a better friend to yourself. You take the very best care of yourself, forever free of waiting until the last minute to finish something. You don't procrastinate anymore.

In your mind you now know, from foundational places deepest inside of you, that you are and you remain a more interested and focused better reader, a voracious reader. A professional Bookworm.

Every book more important, each and every word more interesting and beneficial, you just doing better and better.

Young Adult Moving Forward
Out of School to Career

While you are relaxing floating, drifting, dreaming, and melting into a deeper and deeper state of relaxation right now, you are also treating yourself, better and better, by relaxing beyond both known and as yet unknown to you, any and all barriers, into a brand new and better life a better way of living, a better way of being, while feeling inspired and driven to success in all that you do, all that you are and all that you are now driven to accomplish, while your mind drifts and is actually, whether you realize it or not, drifting, floating and dreaming, while laying the perfectly inspired, foundation for habits and actions that are happily laying the groundwork for a bright and brilliant, self-supportive future.

You let your imagination wander, as if in a dream, and as guided by my voice to a time in the future where you are living on your own and standing on your own 2 feet in your life. At that time you had once long ago, set up the groundwork, goal focused and grew up to make sure we're building a supportive and well-deserved foundation for your life, which has already been done.

A time when you gladly look back upon your past and realize that you are happy that you did the work that was necessary to move forward, achieving the level of success you now enjoy. Once a long time ago, you had been challenged by schoolwork, speed and accuracy, studying to be a *XXXX (client career goal)*.

Although at times the work was slow going and sluggish, and perhaps not as interesting as other things going on around you in your life at the time, there was a point back then when you knuckled down, tightened your belt, and did the work necessary to get the job done to enjoy the safety, the prosperity, the status, recognition and achievement that you now enjoy today.

At that time, you had to set aside some of the fleeting and less important moments, that would stand in the way of the success you now enjoy. From deep inside of you right now you activate the inner wisdom to achieve such a future, a successful and prosperous life, every action, reaction, thought, and feeling, every response, that generates success for this future you, you now to do, and you've drawn toward, because you have unstoppably decided to honor, cherish, nurture and lovingly take care of this future you as necessary, loving yourself completely.

As you relax beyond any and all limits, your mind is now creating successful breakthrough pathways, associations, strategies, and trigger points, both known and unknown to you, which grow stronger, more adaptive, more success oriented, and more precise, to generate greater speed and precision in your technique as a *(XXXX career title)*, finding it all more enjoyable, making time to study and practice, while gaining new perspective in your life.

94

As you react to these things you are unbeatable, as you relax beyond all barriers, you are feeling lighter, better, more guided, flowing in your life, sparkling, in our new harmony of heart and mind, taking even better care of yourself to break yourself through here unbeatably. For what you are doing now, just like maintaining your health, is unbeatably forging your future life, lovingly and respecting and taking the very best care of yourself in the future, and constructing a future in which you are thriving, prosperous, successful, healthy and happy.

It's almost as if the entire world is now working to support you, and encouraging you and cheering you on to success. They want what's best for you, and you generate it and create it, manifesting and creating profound improvement in your life right now, feeling happy excitement, and drive forward toward your goal.

Break-time is over. It is time to seize the moment while creating dramatic success, not because I say so, but because it is the nature of your mind to do this, and to rise above, for the challenge, the minute you are, you remain, and you become, for you believe in yourself, and beyond belief that his faith, and beyond faith is knowing, and you know it is now time to take care, the very best care, of this future you, in ways most appropriate, while standing on your own 2 feet, getting it.

For what the pros know, you know, what they did, you are now doing, how they responded, you respond, and treating this future you like someone you really love and care about, which is only building and building, with precision, intensive speed, almost as if you know what the teachers know.

For the friendships and events that you have right now, will one day be slippery memories from the past, what is more important to you now, and you are more easily able to actively achieve, is focusing on a future, your future, that is bright, financially responsible and supportive, and as much as things can be distracting, you are finding things to be distraction-free about, focused and direct, to support yourself within the kind of a life you now deserve and create unbeatably, you deserve this, and you it now make your own.

Weight Loss & Health

Weight Loss and Emotional Control

You are now certain and sure that you are in a brand new chapter of your life, almost as if someone from deep, deep inside of you, has reset a switch, a dial, a thermostat, or reset a computer of some kind that allows you to be completely satisfied with more moderate meals, less is more, you are filling up sooner, and you are absolutely feeling better.

You are satisfied, you are satiated with food, right now, always, and forever, this time breaking through, always feel full or just even surprisingly satisfied – always enjoying slower placed, properly placed, moderate meals, you now eat slowly, filling up sooner and truly and effectively, even surprisingly feeling filled up and fulfilled in ways both known and unknown to you.

Forever healing, releasing and forgiving whatever caused these situations in the past in your life, or once ever caused you to overeat or feel unsatisfied in anyway.

Certain and sure you are now and remain forever, as a lighter, thinner, breathing easier and healthier, better you, is now unstoppably emerging forever, in the most break-through and complete of ways, not because I say so, but because it is in fact true.

For the greater the challenge, the mightier you become, whether it's stress or anything else, you begin to relax, into a thinner, lighter, better you, almost as if someone has reset your metabolism, as you burn food, fat, weight, calories, in the most un-hungry of ways, feeling fulfilled and satisfied, most effectively, lighter, thinner, healthier and better.

Your correct and ever present response to [stress], is to simply relax, and allow the stress to flow around you, as you find refuge and inner true peace in deep breathing, as wonderful relaxation energy flowing in and out of your heart, in and out of your mind, as you will powerfully rise to the very top, calm, centered and peaceful.

You begin to enjoy moving your body around, standing up, and sitting down, moving from here to there, getting up to get it, getting up to change it, getting up to enjoy your life better, finally and truly getting out of your own way, breaking through here to succeed dramatically, almost as if a heavy burden has been lifted from you, and you have relaxed beyond the limits and barriers, into the very best days and nights, and moments, feelings, thoughts, actions and reactions ahead.

In this brand new and better chapter, you are now eternally hopeful, because truly you know you're breaking through here in the most unlimited of ways right now, as what once seemed too far gone, is now and forever truly with in your grasp, as a lighter, thinner, healthier, longer living, better body it is now attainable, yours on your own, the sweet energy of victory is now yours, for the days of self destructiveness and self-sabotage are now and forever relegated to past moments in your life, now and forever over.

As you watch certain and sure, you are now in a brand new chapter of your life, lighter, thinner, healthier, better, more upbeat, with a can-do attitude, more determined than ever before, activating the energy of every victory, triumph, breakthrough, and success you've ever had, focusing their energies, success limitless, and directing this easily and effectively to shatter and move beyond any and all now and forever vanquished limits that once ever stood in your way, both real and imagined, whether from you or someone else, because you are stepping forward, shedding the past, lighter, thinner healthier and better.

The days and nights of backsliding, have now come to a dramatic end.

Moving unbeatably forward, you redeem and regain your self-respect, you regain a powerfully guided and unstoppable force of success, shining light into the now vanquished shadows from past chapters of your life. For the brightest days in your life now are ahead.

Free Forever of Addictive Binging and Overeating Sweets

You always knew that your life was about to improve, you always knew that habits and issues both known and unknown to you from the past, those that once generated discomfort and disharmony, would in some moment be forever done.

Beginning right now for the rest of your life, in this moment of power, this pivotal point of inspiration, is more solidly yet adaptably yours right now and forever, certain and sure, you are now unbeatable and this, more certain and sure of this than any other time before in your life, because it is so.

In this brand new and better, brighter, more enlightened chapter of your life, which has now begun, your life is now about enjoying yourself and creating a more healthy, happy self, for you have released the past.

You now step boldly into a future where you begin to take better care of yourself, forever free of the things, imbalances, disruptions, upsets, habits, distractions, poor actions, reactions, and discomforts of the past.

By relaxing and slipping forward into this brand new chapter of your life, really and truly feeling and doing great, you have simply grown up a little bit more, leaving your sweet tooth behind, while maintaining the very best happiness and soothing joys of your childhood and life, finding new and better ways of inner and outer fulfillment, using food for nutritional sustenance, finding emotional comfort in healthy choices.

Now being free forever of living to eat, for in this brand new chapter of your life you choose instead to only eat to live, while providing the necessary amounts of healthy food, properly consumed only at mealtimes, food to sustain your body and your life, as your dynamic and always now and forever working in your favor breakthrough, subconscious automatic mind, is instantly, cleverly, and absolutely, working out any and all issues, dynamically and unbeatably in your favor, to break you through forever.

Finding the love and the sweetness in your life, as a small taste of any food slowly savored and melting away in your mouth is enough for you, a small taste and sensation just enough, as you begin to fill up sooner, and actually enjoy the slow savor of one bite, one taste of food.

Free forever and ever of shoveling food down in any way as you are already fulfilled and feeling fine, and free forever of using food ever again to find emotional love and support, as you are now creating newer and better ways of generating that for yourself, the more correct, more fulfilling, and more permanent for you, than ever before.

Inspired truly by the energy of every past victory, triumph and breakthrough you've ever had, or even imagined, as you succeed here and right now, only getting stronger on each and every heartbeat and breath.

You are now feeling wonderfully relaxed, and stress free, having shed the struggle now forever in favor of unstoppable and inspired correct success.

It's almost as if someone from deep, deep inside of you, as reset a as switch, a dial, thermostat, or a powerful and absolute computer of some kind, substantially and forever, dynamically and effectively, fluidly and adaptably, working any and all of this out for you, in ways so healthy, the very best just for you.

Ahhh, it feels great to be so free.

Growing up into this new chapter of your life and seizing your power both inner and outer, you liberate your mighty inner hero, the part of you that is doubtless and fearless, focused and unbeatable, the part that is mighty and unstoppable, rising up and becoming mightier than any of those things, to break you through here forever and unbeatably, and so it is, and so remains now and forever.

Your mind and your body, even your emotions and your thoughts, work in harmony and concert, in ways most effective, truly finding comfort, serenity, and peace, to binge no more, now forever done, shoved into the past, you know certain and sure, now free forever.

In the past may have been things that you felt drove you crazy, but in this brand new inspiring unbeatable chapter of your life, the energy of all of those past imbalances now are restructured, to fortify you, strengthen you, make you pull you together mightily, in the ways that are very best and most supportive to you.

So certain here and now, having done the work automatically and effectively, relaxation focused, as you are relaxing deeper and further, you seem as if you are relaxing into eight to twelve years worth of healing, each and every time you do this on your own, pulling your success together amazingly, any and all of this getting stronger and better for you.

You are remaining withdrawal symptom free, craving free, feeling whole and wonderful, together, fulfilled and satisfied, instinctively and automatically making better choices for yourself, as a new foundation in your life is now enhanced and set forth into effective unstoppable action.

A small taste is now enough, you eat in designated eating areas only, free of any distractions, smaller plates, less is more, healthy food choices, fruits, vegetables, lean meats, whole grains, you fill up and are fulfilled sooner, in proper proportions, taking the very best care of yourself.

Each and every step that is success, leading to grander and greater successes and steps into a brighter and better future, reorganized and unlimited, cleverly and dynamically creating ways for you to succeed, in spite of and most especially because of the past as you now rise up, beyond the past, and because of the past, you are forever freed.

You now focus upon the present, creating a better future for yourself with every bite, making healthy choices, always remaining in complete control, experiencing simple satisfaction with smaller, apprpriate portions.

Your new label, is unaddicted, freed, safe, healthy, mighty, liberated, blockage free, improved in the ways that matter most to you, now free.

You easily and dynamically achieve self-discipline. Rather than struggling, you let go, you relax, you thrive, and even find passionate reasons, thoughts, feelings, ideas, even excuses, as you are and as you remain.

You now relaxed and safe, doing just fine, amazing and impressing everyone, most especially yourself, as an extension of yourself, and you found love for yourself and your life, that you now generate.

With each and every breath and each and every beat of your heart, while you are awake, while you are asleep, even while your deep and powerful, pleasant dreams work this out for you.

Overcoming Sugar Cravings

As you relax, float, drift, and dream, you have relaxed your your way barrier free, into a barrier free life. Taking better care of yourself, all things that once stood and your way, are and remain no longer.

In fact, it may even feel to you, almost as if, a light from on high has shown down upon you, or washing away and vanquishing any and all shadows, or maybe instead, someone, from deep, deep inside of you, has reset a switch, a dial, a computer, or a thermostat of some kind, allowing release, dynamic healing, forgiveness, as you re-coalesce while finding better balance in your life, loving yourself enough to heal, better encouraged now, thrive and succeed, almost as if been born anew, yet doing even better this time.

In this moment, you truly and significantly embrace your mighty inner hero, wiser and respectful of the fact that you have stood mightily, through great challenges, knowing you will always be able to do the same, just as you have always done, and now forever shall do and remain.

More and more, you are inspired, yet even driven, to do things that work for you to improve your body and your life, in your favor, including, following your life improvement program, while reducing sugar intake.

Your mind, in ways both known and unknown to you, begins to work this out and rectify all imbalances, while generating balance, peace, harmony, a mighty can-do spirit.

You now begin to realize that a small taste of any food now savored in a small portioned amount, is enough for you, taking better care of yourself while extending your longevity, with less sugar, it's useless, no longer wanted, no longer needed, and less junk food.

Foods in this new chapter you have in fact, truly, outgrown, always free forever of using food as a reward.

In this brand new, better, more and more successful and fluidly effective, chapter of your life, you eat to live, rather than living to eat.

Food from childhood years, now left behind, more and more, outgrown, undesirable, now more and more unappealing, whether it be *ice cream, cheese doodles, chocolate, hot chocolate*, or anything else, is best left in the past.

You have moved on in ways that take better care of you, automatically, in ways known and unknown to you.

Seizing the moment, and relaxing barrier free, forward into your life, keeping things in moderation, new disciplines are easy, automatic reactions begin to manifest and gestate.

You even seem to now like [eating raw food], preparing what you buy, natural foods, whole foods, vegetables, best prepared in your favor to take better care of yourself.

Body, emotions, mind whole, healing better, harmony, taking better care of you.

Necessary and desirable regiments, easily taking supplements in a timely way, it's all taken in stride, so free and automatic, in order for you,to do better, in order to thrive, staying strong as needed, spending as necessary, always free of spending unnecessarily, you save more and feel fine, inside and out, both day and night.

Overcoming Carbs and Exercising More

In this new and better chapter of your life, you choose to eat better, healthy, sensible, more moderate, and life-supporting foods and meals each and every time you decide to eat to sustain your body and your life.

You choose to increase your protein, while reducing your carbohydrates.

Your first, best natural response, is to choose protein over carbohydrates anytime you need to eat, enjoying your breakfast better with a higher protein ratio while eating slowly, sensibly, slowly chewing your food, knowing when enough is enough, knowing when to stop, you are already full.

Smaller plates, eating only in designated eating areas, free of media distractions like television.

Eating times are times of relaxation and nutrition, calmness and inner and outer peace.

When you get too hungry, a protein-based snack is so much better for you.

You know, it's amazing, how easy it is to choose protein over carbohydrates, your tastes, habits, actions and reactions all re-tuned, reset and recalibrated in your favor to succeed here.

When having a snack, a bite or two is enough for you.

A small taste and sensation, is enough to satisfy and satiate, choosing to front load the bulk of your food, eating earlier and filling up sooner, you now so much more full and fulfilled late at night.

More and more free from and not into the foods, cookies, cake, which often, just a mouthful or instead, just a small taste, is enough for you.

You begin to treat yourself in a more self loving way, most especially when it comes to eating, you treating yourself like an adult does, sustaining your life and taking better care of your health through proper fulfillment and nutrition.

A small taste of anything, is enough to knock out your desire for it, and to completely fill you up.

For the greater the challenge, the mightier you become, in this brand new and better chapter of your life.

You bring your exercise goals down to levels of ridiculous ease, finding reasons even excuses, even finding supportive friends, helping you enjoy the gym and better exercise. Your mind is automatically, instantly, and profoundly working any and all of this out in your favor unbeatably, in ways both known and unknown to you, it all just seems to be happening for you.

I wonder if you even get realize how truly easy this is for you to break through thrive and succeed here, the weight just seems to be melting off, with each and every action, each and every reaction, each and every breath, each and every heartbeat.

Any and all of this, easily, thrivingly succeeding or simply melting off 10, 18, 26, 37, 38, even 41 pounds, as a newer, lighter, healthier, better you now emerges.

Ahhhh, it feels so great to be so light and so free, happy and knowing you can!

Weight Loss with Divine Support

It's almost as if someone from deep, deep inside of you has reset a switch, a dial, a computer or a thermostat of some kind that restores and balances your body, calms you, soothes you, releases and relieve any and all of your stress, resets, and balances the fluids of the body, even all that is your hormones are now functioning in better balance and in restorative ways, both known and unknown to you.

Less is more, you fill up sooner, eating only free of media distractions like television.

You learn to savor the taste of food in your mouth, so even a small taste of bread, pasta, rice and potatoes, just a small taste and sensation of sweet, pastries, completely fulfills your need for sensation, you get the complete and necessary sensation, as a mouthful is enough to satisfy you in ways so very complete.

You learn to take enjoyment in movement, almost as if the way you used to exercise, is now the way you do.

A new chapter of your life has begun, you're more energetic, and filled with vitality, so re-tuned, reset, recalibrated, your mighty inner hero, now rising to the top, finding better ways to thrive and succeed, automatically, in ways known and unknown to you.

Proper portions in balance and in harmony, fill you up sooner, as you eat more slowly, knowing when enough is enough.

Relaxed right now and relaxing deeper, all that you are, body, emotions, mind, even spirit, memorizes this feeling of deep relaxation and is now more enabled to come right back to this very place if not deeper, anytime you need to, after just a few deep breaths, finding calm this, peace, and stillness, more easily able to get back here whenever you need to.

Eating slowly, smaller portions, on smaller plates, dishes, and bowls, one portion, contained within those containers contents you, making you feel fulfilled, for enough is enough, just right and fulfilling for you.

Regardless if you're feeling wonderful, and centered, peaceful, calm, or stressed out and filled with anxiety, in this brand new and better chapter of your life, you are taking better care of yourself and loving yourself better, free of ever eating food again without thinking.

As you have relaxed barrier-free into the very best moments of the new life you are building for yourself, in this polished, shiny, a new chapter of your life, so much more right for you, you are confident, clear, sharp, and trusting in your life as you have now a higher metabolism, burning food, weight, calories, in ways so right and so wonderful, just for you.

In this newer, better, brighter, more life-supporting chapter, more unlimited, more empowered, more inspired, you begin to create a better dream of a life.

Each and every thought, each and every action, each and every reaction, fortifies and strengthens you, builds a higher wisdom and inner strength, as you are now more than ever completely ready, with each and every breath, and with each and every heartbeat.

You now embrace the powerful yet every day idea, that all in your life that changes will only be a you improvement and strength, wisdom and guidance, and better fulfillment, in each and every moment, feeling brighter, shinier and newer.

Not only is God now willing, following inner and outer guidance as well as Guidance from on high, you make time to be calm and find balance, and listen to your guidance, and now not only simply feel fulfilled, but also, lighter and enlightened, to embrace that wisdom eternal and profound guidance and now, while completely out of your own way, readily embrace such guidance, blending with it and becoming truly at one with it, all and any of it, only the very best, now a part of you and your own, the very best now like sun shining down from someplace above, now your very own.

Free of Late Night Eating, Meal Pacing

By relaxing beyond any and all old barriers, as you have relaxed beyond all limits and habits, into a better rhythm and pace in your life, more easily supporting each and every thought, to allow better moments in your existence to breakthrough here.

You choose to eat larger meals earlier in the day, finding a different pace, while remaining completely un-hungry and satisfied and even satiated, right through and into the next morning, most especially at night.

Each and every bedtime, each and every evening, you are powerfully free of eating or wanting to eat or craving anything to eat because moderately paced, more fulfilling meals consumed earlier in the day are more satisfying, more correct, and more appropriate for you.

You have decided to take better care of yourself, eating a fairly reasonable breakfast, a larger lunch, and a moderate dinner, that allows you to achieve your goals with ease, not because I say so, but because it is now the nature of your own mind, in this brand new and better chapter of your life, that allows you to love and take better care of yourself, eating moderately, on and off as needed, remaining uncommonly un-hungry and fulfilled, while relaxing beyond, over, and through, any and all old barriers that ever stood in your way .

You choose to eat most of your food intake during the day, taking any and all necessary measures to move you forward into a more comfortable rhythm at night, one in which your stomach is calm and peaceful.

Deep and soothing breathing guides your way, beyond today's possibly stressful patterns, becoming stress-free at night, unwinding, while allowing yourself a calm and comfortable stomach, and a wonderful soothing peaceful night of rest.

Each and every night at bedtime, you'll enjoy reinforcing all of this, using relaxation techniques, as well as putting the entire day's worth of thoughts, actions, emotions, feelings, anticipations, and even the ideas, on the shelf, one to two hours before bedtime, allowing your body, your emotions, your mind, and even your spirit, to relax into a brand new harmony, that allows you to thrive while remaining fulfilled, filled up, satiated, and ready to unwind comfortably, sleeping right through the night, as if you were once again a child, turning into bed at night, ready to sleep, relax, and float into a place of happy, supportive, even fun, encouraging dreams.

All of this not because I say so, but because it is the nature of your own mind to do so, and you're already there, for each and every time you repeat this wonderfully enjoyable technique on your own, you relax a deeper, quicker, more effectively, for the greater the barriers once were, the mightier and better, even more effective you are.

You take and make the time to love yourself, to take better care of yourself, to treat yourself like someone you care about, to set aside to time to eat slowly, calmly, for in fact truly, you're eating times now become about, and remain about, a time of calm. peacefulness, and a time of sustenance, in which you fulfilling yourself physically, to sustain your vitality, health, and longevity, relaxing your emotions to take better care of yourself, unwinding your thoughts as your mind now clears and as your thoughts eventually clear and amazingly sharp, directed, focused, goal directed and focused, even solution-oriented, completely allowing you greater focus, tranquility and breakthrough, thriving success, in truly inspired and unbeatable ways.

Once in awhile at night, just a small bite, one fork-full, one spoon-full, or a small taste is enough for you. One bite, one taste, that you savor in your mouth only for a taste, you are both now and forever truly finding complete fulfillment.

You find any and all of this not only calming, but now you know better - you've had enough, and right then and there, you're done.

As you are practically eating nothing at night from here on out, as you are feeling hunger-free, fulfilled, and satisfied in surprisingly effective an adaptive flourishing ways of achieving optimum results both known and unknown to you, it feels great to be so free.

Less is more, you are filling up sooner. You have reinvented the way you are going about sustaining yourself, to take the very best care of yourself. In these moments of deep and soothing, truly rejuvenating and life renovating relaxation, your objectives and powerful dynamic subconscious mind are now truly releasing, forgiving, and moving beyond the thoughts, experiences, actions, reactions, and misinterpretations of the past, to break you through here unbeatably.

In fact, you've relaxed your way into a brand new and better, happier and lighter, better chapter of your life, feeling a new sense of seizing the moment while being completely in control of your life, and your urges, have lost power and control over your life and most especially anything to do with food.

Free forever you are and you remain of over eating simply because food is there. You are taking so much better care of yourself now, in this lighter, thinner, healthier, and better chapter of your life, than ever before.

Your clever, always working in your favor, adaptive mind, is now creating a moment of pause and realization within you that allows you to break free forever from patterns of the past, from right now, old and finished past chapters of your life, are now done, as you are now and powerfully remain instead where you wanted to be, should be and now firmly, adaptively, cleverly and creatively are - now focused on savoring just a small taste, rather than eating without tasting, just a small taste, even one bite, is enough for you.

This makes you feel wonderful, and you are wonderful, as your mighty inner hero is now activated, working only in your favor to powerfully break you free. You are powerfully successful and free of being overly hungry, overeating, or craving anything, simply feeling content and comfortable, even un-hungry, even when challenged.

You are now creating, manifesting and replacing the old ways to better deal with your emotions in a more balanced and harmonized way, determined to rise above and finding better ways to live your life more enjoyably and upbeat.

In a previous chapter of your life, you may have eaten or not eaten just for various reasons, but now in this new, better, improved more success oriented chapter of your life, you are finding every reason while adaptively creating better reasons to become and forever remain lighter, healthier, thinner, and better, creating reasons, reactions, thoughts, feelings and adaptations and even more especially better ways to feel fulfilled, calm and centered, inside you.

You now, serene, as a sea of tranquility, with a healthier and higher metabolism, better taste, better placed, easily moderated, as if you're working with a coach to correct this, from deep, deep inside of you, as you are releasing un-needed, forgiven, released, and seemingly melting away any and all old habits that ever stood and your way, and it feels great to be free of those imbalances, now that you are truly powerful.

In fact, every time you relax like this, most especially right now, it is almost as if someone from deep, deep inside of you has reset a switch, the dial, the thermostat, or set into motion a computer of some kind, which is easily allowing you to break through here unbeatably.

Imagine now any success you've ever had magnified by 80,000 times, all of that breakthrough energy and encouragement, inspiration, and drive, determination and ability to succeed, all around you right now and forever. You are now certain, serene and sure that you are now and forever powerfully free of any and all old urges that ever once stood in your way, both known and unknown to you, as you are so very easily and successfully moving on, having gained power and control over your life and your body and most especially easily succeeding and triumphing over anything to do with food.

In fact, you've relaxed into a brand new and better, happier and lighter better chapter of your life, feeling a new sense of being completely in control of your life and your body, in control of your urges, completely freed from the past and in a brighter, better, lighter, thinner, healthier chapter of your life.

You are powerfully successful and free of being overly hungry, most especially finding better ways of dealing with stress, like detaching yourself from the moment, while deep breathing, calming down, feeling better, free forever of ever using food as a crutch to deal with stress.

In fact, you've relaxed your way into a brand new and better, happier and lighter, better chapter of your life, feeling a new sense of seizing the moment while being completely in control of your life, and your urges, having gained power and control over your life and most especially while easily overwhelming in your favor, anything to do with food.

Free Forever of Addictive Caffeine and Sugar Eating

You always knew that your life was about to improve, you always knew that habits and issues both known and unknown to you from the past, that once generated discomfort and disharmony, would in some moment be forever done.

So surely beginning right now for the rest of your life, in this moment of power, this pivotal point of inspirational power, is more solidly yet adaptably yours right now and forever, certain and sure, you are now unbeatable and this, more certain and sure of this than any other time before in your life, because it is so.

In this brand new and better, brighter, more enlightened, and just doing better, chapter of your life, which has now and forever begun, your life is now about enjoying yourself, as you have released the past.

As you now step boldly into a future where you begin to take better care of yourself, for gone now and forever of the things, imbalances, disruptions, upsets, habits, actions, reactions, and discomforts of the past.

Your energy just right, your life is sweet enough; you are fulfilled and refreshed, just doing fine.

By relaxing and slipping forward into this brand new chapter of your life, really and truly feeling and doing great, you have simply grown up a little bit more, while maintaining the very best happiness and soothing joys of your childhood and life.

You are finding new and better ways of inner and outer fulfillment, while being free forever of old ways and patterns, breaking through here and forever releasing old cycles that are no longer life sustaining and supportive, now only life supporting habits and cycles see you through, you are drawn to them and they are now one with you.

You are now feeling fine and automatically doing better, even if you have yet to realize it, taking better and better care of yourself, eating to live, more and more caffeine free, sugar free.

Old ways and addictions, unravel, evaporate, just fizzle out, your dynamic mind just working things out in your favor.

All of this rendering you calm, peaceful, very flexible, all re-tuned and reset, just doing fine.

For in this brand new chapter of your life you choose to only <u>eat to live</u>, new ways, better foods, better nights even better days, now guide your way, while providing the necessary amounts of food, properly consumed only at mealtimes, food to sustain your body and your life.

Drawn to better, doing great, even best, as your dynamic and always now and forever working in your favor breakthrough, subconscious automatic mind, is instantly, cleverly, and absolutely, working out any and all issues, dynamically in your favor, in ultimately effective ways, both known and unknown to you.

Finding the sweetness in your life, as a small taste of any food slowly savored and melting away in your mouth is enough for you, a small taste and sensation just enough, as you begin to fill up sooner, and actually enjoy the slow savor of one taste of food, free forever of ever shoveling food down in any way, as you are already fulfilled and feeling fine.

Free forever of using food ever again to find emotional love and support, as you are now creating newer and better ways of generating that for yourself the more correct, more fulfilling, and more permanent for you, than ever before.

Inspired truly by the energy of every past victory, triumph and breakthrough you've ever had, or even imagined, as you succeed here and right now, only getting stronger on each and every heartbeat and breath, as you are now feeling wonderfully relaxed, and stress free, having shed the struggle now forever in favor of unstoppable and inspired correct success.

It's almost as if someone from deep, deep inside of you, as reset a as switch, a dial, thermostat, or a powerful and absolute computer of some kind, substantially and forever, dynamically and effectively, fluidly and adaptably, working any and all of this out for you, in ways so healthy, the very best just for you.

Ahhhhh, it feels great to be so free.

Growing up into this new chapter of your life and seizing your power both inner and outer, you liberate your mighty inner hero, the part of you that is doubtless and fearless, focused and unbeatable, the part that is mighty and unstoppable, rising up and becoming mightier than any of those things, to break you through here forever, and so it is, and so remains now and forever.

Your mind and your body, even your emotions and your thoughts, work in harmony and concert, to break you through here fluidly and comfortably, in ways most effective, truly finding comfort, serenity, and peace.

Mindlessly eating or even any bingeing, now heroically defeated, completely let go of, released, now forever done, shoved into the past, floating and flowing away, you know so, very certain and sure, you now free forever.

In the past there may have been things that you felt drove you crazy, but in this brand new inspiring unbeatable chapter of your life, the energy of all of those past imbalances, now are restructured, to fortify you, strengthen you, make you pull you together mightily, and to powerfully and effectively break you through here honestly, and in the ways that are very best and most supportive to you.

Certainly here and now, having done the work automatically and effectively, relaxation focused, as you are relaxing deeper and further, you seem as if you are relaxing into eight to twelve years worth of automatic healing each and every time you do this on your own.

Pulling your success together amazingly, any and all of this getting stronger and better for you, you are remaining, withdrawal symptom free, craving free, feeling whole and wonderful, together, fulfilled, even maybe serene, and enough, instinctively and automatically making better choices for yourself, as a new foundation in your life is now enhanced and set forth into effective unstoppable action.

Enough is enough, you having now had enough, you eat in designated eating areas only, free of media distractions like the tevision, better actions, better reactions to yourself and the world around you.

Less is more, you fill up and are fulfilled sooner, in proper proportions, taking the very best care of yourself, just like an unconditionally loving parent would correctly treat and love, exceptionally wonderful and beautiful child, you now truly know that child, healed and whole, taking the very best care of yourself, each and every step that is success, leading to grander and greater successes and steps into a brighter and better future.

Reorganized and unlimited, cleverly and dynamically creating ways for you to succeed at this, in spite of and most especially because of the past as you now rise up, beyond the past, and because of the past, you're forever freed, you're now focused upon the present, creating a better future for yourself.

Taking the label off yourself, your new label, is unaddicted, freed, safe, healthy, mighty, liberated, blockage free, improved in the ways that matter most to you, now free.

You easily and dynamically achieve the discipline, at this time.

Rather than struggling, you let go, you relax, you thrive, and even find passionate reasons, thoughts, feelings, ideas, even excuses, as you are and as you remain, breaking through right here, for more than a small taste, totally unappealing.

You now relaxed and safe, doing just fine, amazing and impressing everyone, most especially yourself, as an extension of yourself and you found love for yourself and your life, that you now generate.

Any and all of this working out for you and each and every moment of your life, with each and every breath and on each and every beat of your heart, while you are awake, while you are asleep, even while your deep and powerful, pleasant dreams work this out for you.

114

For the greater the resistance, the mightier and more dynamically unstoppable you become, while you are awake, while you were asleep, even what you dream at night, peacefully, at the end fulfilling dreams, now out of your way, unblocked, free, doing better, more certain and sure of this than any other time before in your life.

Weight Management – for Busy Professionals

You are released, you are healed, you are forgiven of past critical self-judgments, while relaxing beyond all barriers into a brand new chapter of your life.

For it is time to succeed here, and breakthrough, as never before.

In fact you are doing 90,000 times better than you have ever imagined possible, not because I say so, but because you have made an important decision to move forward into a brand new chapter of your life, and so it is, and so it remains, and you even feel this and know it to be true.

You are substantially motivated to cleverly and adaptably achieve a lighter, thinner, and healthier better you, in highly effective ways, most meaningful, even more effectively, especially whenever challenged by feelings, thoughts, actions, and reactions, from previous chapters of your life.

Any and all of these just getting easier, more adaptive, and more cleverly precise, most especially during any moment when you might be stressed, whether at work, or with family and or social situations where you are now effectively choosing to breathe deep and soothing, steadying breath, which calms you down, balances you, while you are generating a new sense of security and serenity.

Remaining calm, balanced, comfortable, centered, even re-identified, within a brand new chapter of your life, finding comfort, feeling self-assured, remaining centered, while trusting in the vital fact that all previous moments of your life have in some way supported you.

You are now using this unstoppable force of energy and inspiration to support yourself in even better ways, knowing that this moment is a place of power and foundational strength, serenity, gentleness and ease, you now, more easily rising to the top more *especially* whenever challenged.

Each and every thought, each and every feeling, each and every action and reaction, which you are choosing to experience and embrace, activate or make real, is being directed by your powerful mind to allow you enhanced feelings of self support, any time of day, evenings, mornings or [most especially in the middle part of the afternoon at work].

Even if your physical and emotional energy level is low and or you've already seen a number of clients/patients, you instead and even better, are feeling fine, and rising to the top, just as you have done at numerous other times before, you steadily succeeding here, lighter, thinner, healthier, less is more, you are filling up sooner, with a higher metabolism, burning food, fat, weight and calories more efficiently and effectively than ever before.

You are just taking better care of yourself, less is more, one very small taste is enough for you, most especially during [6-7 PM] when you leave work but can not go directly home because there might be some scheduled evening obligation... either more work, or a meeting of some kind.

You have in fact, relaxed beyond any and all barriers, into a brand new chapter of your life, all of this just getting easier and better, most especially whenever you are or might be, driving to work in the morning. . . particularly [on mornings when you attend meetings], allowing a more balanced and upbeat you to emerge.

Just as with times in the past, you're allowing yourself to put the day that you just experienced on the shelf, while your breathing becomes steadier and more calm, more relaxing, at bedtime, where you just simply, put your head on the pillow, close your eyes, and go to sleep, just as you've done, thousands of times before, you are allowing your bedtime to become a happier, more and better rewarding, a place a personal rejuvenation, while remaining free of overheating, even perhaps enjoying a couple of cool glasses of filling, fulfilling, flourishing water before bedtime.

It's really becoming wonderfully easy for you to knock off and relax at bedtime, healing, so very drowsy, so very weary, so easily able to unwind as your thoughts become pleasantly cloudy and so very calm, so very relaxed, a better you now emerging effectively, even enjoying self-hypnotic reinforcement as all of you seems to be melting away any and all thoughts and cares, as all of you unwinds and relaxes.

You simply just put your head down on the pillow, close your eyes and easily and deeply fall asleep, just as you have done 10,000's of times in the past.

Any and all of this, becoming more clever, easy, effective and adaptive.

You are truly finding newer and better ways to effectively rise above any and all stressful challenges from the past, while becoming stress-free, content, all of this more adaptable and easy for you.

You may even feel in fact that you are effectively releasing any and all old stressors that in the now done, old and now forever finished, previous chapters of your life which had caused you to feel insecure or vulnerable, for you now, bound and determined.

You are able to rise above any and all challenges presented, for the truth is, has always been and shall ever remain, you are always rising to the top while confidently and skillfully dealing with challenges presented, however in this brand new chapter of your life it's becoming easier and more methodical, more skillful and effective, even while or most especially when emotionally challenged, you now are just doing better and better, easily and adaptively *avoiding food as a crutch* within your life, whatever the energy demands upon you, now and forever, better.

And instead, you are abundant energetically and rising to the top, forever free of destructive patterns, forever *freed of binge eating,* forever free of the minute details that stood in your way, as you now are succeeding on the deepest and truest levels of life.

As your mighty inner hero is activated, and is effectively working in your favor, while you're awake, while you are asleep, even while you're dreaming, cleverly and adaptively working out new strategies for greater success, free of overdoing anything, as you are and you remain lighter, thinner, healthier, better, most especially while presenting, taking care of family situations, whatever the energy demand, you now with boundless and unstoppable energy, getting through, breaking through, deep breathing relaxation breath.

If challenged by any project, whether ahead or behind, feeling pleased with yourself, inspired and able, enabled, loving yourself better, free of old habits and patterns, free of any need to overdo things, free of craving carbohydrates uselessly, less is more, you are feeling fulfilled inside and out, as your emotions balance, your mind clears, you drink plenty of life giving water, while taking things in a new stride, so self-supporting, and stress-free.

Healing and Empowerment
for Illness Freedom

Demanding a higher light that will enliven your body, you allow, create, demand and call forth, and so there is now, as if, a beam shimmering and iridescent golden-white light now flows down from above and all around you and embraces your skin, completely vanquishing and thoroughly eliminating any and all imbalance and shadow.

Light vanquishes shadow, you know this, your truth, while healing and reorganizing, restoring, making as new, any and all tissue, blood, bone, muscle, organ, connective tissue, as you now and forever move into a brand new chapter of your life while you realize and recognize, that you are meant to be here, feeling comfortable and happy, knowing that you are embraced and surrounded by a healing and glistening light.

As you are relaxed, your heart opens up like a giant flower now, self-assuredly feeling so loved, so a part of the human race, truly knowing right now you are so better off in this place of refuge and healing, experiencing an energy and healing upgrade right now, so easily remembered as you are being restored, that you are very likely to come back to this place for an even higher upgrade on a regular basis, for more of the same.

As you relax, you become rejuvenated, in fact are rejuvenated in complete ways, both known and unknown to you as you relax, relaxation brining inner and outer peace, tranquility, calmness, and truest and highest Divinely inspired healing, feeling and knowing the power of your relaxation the power of your breath, as it is and remains with every wave of energy bringing deeper healing and relaxation.

The fog completely lifts, your mind now clears, as your ability to visualize now becomes a optimized, simply by relaxing, all of you is unfolding and opening like a flower.

Your mind now clear and free, empowered and inspired, you now more easily and readily manifest everything and anything that you put your mind to, generating a powerful wave of unstoppable healing abundance while overcoming.

You now the mighty one, truly and thoroughly healing well, rising up in wholeness and balance, supporting yourself in the very best ways, and the very most complete of ways, spiritually, mentally, emotionally, even physically, a new harmony of self, knitting you back together again as you manifest into your life by relaxing.

Opening your mind now, calling fourth, summoning forth, everything and anything you need, including improved behavior, in order to be in every moment, even while thinking we're simply going through the days of your life, in order to be taking the very best care of yourself, generating proper nutritional habits, eating the right foods, allowing your body to heal, while easily able to generate optimal improvement in your life.

Ready to take this on, feeling a new serene sensibility and a peace inside and out of you, multiplying and healing you, as you feel the love, as you love and are more noticeably lovable, generating peace inside and out, rising up to become mighty, heroically breaking through, supporting yourself in profoundly new and better ways.

Each and every aspect, working in harmony and concert, healing yourself, truly healing yourself, relinquishing fear, rising up, becoming mighty and heroic, truly an unstoppable force in your life, with single minded focus to generate healing and balance, strength and serenity, peace and love, as your inner child now at peace, love and supported, easily able to generate what you need, while the light all around you, generates unstoppable healing, vanquishing any and all old shadows, activating and sparking your immune system, almost as if, someone from deep, deep inside of you, has reset a switch, or activated a dial, computer, or reset a thermostat of some kind, that allows you to break through shamelessly and mightily.

Your life begins to reorganize, your thoughts and experiences, now activate your inner fighter, to fight unbeatably and unstoppably driven, to accept nothing less than success and healing, balance and restoration, empowerment and strength, and every aspect of your life, while loving yourself enough to do this and generate exceptional results, in ways both known and unknown to you, as you rise up and become fearlessly heroic to fight imbalance, restore harmony and generate balance, to vanquished any and all lack, while manifesting the truest and most flowing abundance, feeling a new sense of inner and outer love, which becomes a magnet for all things wonderful and better in your life.

Ahh, you now restored, you now loved, you now mighty, you now taking better care of yourself, eating properly, released and restored and relaxed, doing better and better, taking the very best care of yourself, all of this moving forward in ways both known and unknown, taking the very best care of yourself, and even occasionally surprised at how easy and forever this becomes.

Weight Extras 1

You are now and forever remain cleverly and adaptive, completely effective at this, even in surprising ways.

By eating smaller meals consistently throughout the day, at nighttime you are powerfully free of ever late-night snacking, but even if you did, a small taste would be enough for you, you have moved on into a brighter, better, healthier, lighter, thinner, better chapter of your life.

Less is more, you have filled up sooner, just a small taste is enough to satisfy a sensation or feeling you may need.

In this new improved chapter of your life, a mouthful or perhaps just a sensation on your tongue is enough, free forever you are and you remain of overdoing ice cream, cake, or fruits, in fact any sweets at all, a small taste is enough, as you enjoy the privilege of the sensation better with just a small taste rather than flooding yourself as it once was in previous now done chapters of your life.

Just a small taste of carbs, a small bite of bread, taste or two of pasta, the sensation of something sweet, a sip of a drink, are all enough for you, anything more is less than pleasant, you already are fulfilled, you're satisfied, you are satiated, you are fulfilled.

Mealtimes, free of media distractions like television, but off a smaller plate, slowly consumed, make you feel better about yourself and your life.

Smaller portions eaten more slowly, derive better nutrition for you in the most very beneficial of ways, taking care of you in the very best of ways.

In fact, you may just find, you are cleverly adapting all that you do, say, think, feel, and react to, in surprisingly effective breakthrough ways, or perhaps you are simply to succeeding at this brilliantly, feeling so very energetically inspired by every past victory, triumph, breakthrough, and success you've ever had.

Your new point of view and experience is about eating only when you are hungry, or at proper mealtimes paced safely and smartly throughout the day, as the weight just seems to be melting from your body, and you thrive, polished by the experience into a lighter, thinner, better you.

Each little step forward meaning a lot. You imagine and visualize yourself at the right size, the right weight, and your mind's image helps you to generate the body and feelings you pleasurably need and achieve.

You relax and have completely stepped forward into a brand new chapter of your life, seizing the moment while cleverly and adaptively creating a more-healthy lifestyle where you eat better while extending your health, your life, your longevity, while maintaining wonderful energy.

You make, find, and create time to exercise, just a few minutes that you grab, at the just right comfortable time of day, so right for you, which the easily spills over into an enjoyable program as any and all additional weight just seems to be melting off your body, not because they say so, it's just that your metabolism is actually going up, and up, almost as if someone, from deep, deep inside of you, has reset a switch, and dial, computer, or a thermostat of some kind, easily allowing food, fat, weight, and calories, to be burned from your body easily and effectively, and almost amazing ways.

As if someone has forever activated your self-control switch, as you relax beyond any and all old barriers, into the very best chapter of your life, seizing the moment, completely in control of your actions, habits, desires, any and all of those working completely within your favor, all the while feeling hunger-free and satisfied.

All of this is both now and forever energizing you and inspiring you to greater levels of success.

In this brand new chapter of your life however, you begin to take better care of yourself, a small taste is just enough for you, to satisfy and satiate any and all urges you once had from previous chapters of your life, as those old urges seem to be fading into the past far, far away from you.

You grow up, free of overdoing the food, taking the very best care of yourself, making healthy food choices, receiving proper nutrition.

You choose to eat in designated eating areas, far away from media distractions like television, while well paced, relaxed, calm, and comfortable, off smaller plates, less is more, you fill up sooner, your metabolism is higher and better, just right for you, and more rejuvenating to you.

In the evening, you calm down, your body, emotions, mind, in fact all that you are, are comfortable and peaceful late night, choosing instead to drink plenty of life giving water in the evening washing you clean inside, as your hunger seems to fade with every sip.

In this new chapter of your life, you are free of eating food ever again without thinking, even if it's just in front of you and most especially if you're not hungry or have had enough to eat throughout the day to sustain your life and body.

Even when you can't stick to a diet, you are doing fine, smaller portions of better, more healthy food and greater energy rule the day and the night as you become lighter, thinner, healthier and better.

It's amazing to notice, how easy it is for you to win by releasing and resolving from your body, 7, 12, 18, 23, 24, 26, even 31 pounds.

You only eat when you need to, eating to sustain your life, having grown up and you are now taking better care of yourself.

You are powerfully free of eating or wanting to eat or craving anything to eat just because food is around.

You only eat when you need to, eating healthy foods in proper portions to sustain life, health, and limitless vitality, having grown up and you are now taking better care of yourself.

You choose to eat only when necessary, you only eat when you are hungry, gone now and forever are the days and shoveling food down, in this brave new and better chapter of your life, you take a small taste, allow it to melt in your mouth, whether it's sweets or anything else 'taboo' and savoring the sensations, tastes and aromas, as just a small taste is enough for you.

You're powerfully successful and free of kiddy foods, now that you are an adult, you prefer fruits and vegetables and lean meats over sugary carbs.

You relax and you allow your mind to wander now, relaxing ever deeper, and begin to recalibrate the way you are thinking about eating, viewing what you eat, automatically just doing better for yourself, as it's now and forever okay to leave some of each and every meal on the plate, eating off a smaller dish, choosing to eat only in areas that are designated for food, chewing and eating slowly, free of media distractions like television, filling up sooner, less is more, as you become lighter, thinner, healthier and better.

As you relax beyond the old limits into a brand new, exciting and more robust chapter of your life, you are creatively exploring, maintaining, in creating better portion control and knowing when you are full, not because I say so, but because it's the nature of your own mind and dynamic spirit to arrange this, in ways both known and unknown to you, and so it is and remains forever.

Different foods now more appealing to you, including your new found desire for more salads and whole grains.

You allow your imagination to wander further now creating a strong and powerful image of who you are in the present moment, more easily burning off weight, food, fat, and calories, food more easily burned off your body, generating a wonderful present appearance.

You are powerfully free of eating or wanting to eat or craving anything to eat just because you are or might be stressed, bored, or while feeling any other emotional response.

You imagine now and see, and generate, from your thoughts, and your emotions, your very best weight, [155 pounds], as 17, 26, 38, or even 39lbs. seems to be melting away into now done and past chapters of your life as you're feeling fantastic and on top of the world.

In this brand new and better chapter of your life, your eating times now and forever become and steadfastly remain, about the sustenance, so you slow down, chew your food more completely, savoring and taking the time necessary to enjoy your meal and digest properly taking better care of yourself here, automatically, in ways both known and unknown to you.

Smaller portions or a small taste of food intended for children, like kiddy food or junk food, is enough to satisfy any and all cravings, as you allow the taste to melt in your mouth, you choose to know when enough is enough, you had enough, and it is done, as a newer, lighter, less hungry, more sustained, and fulfilled you, emerges unbeatably.

You begin to eat in a healthy regimen, pacing your meals throughout the day, three meals a day, five smaller meals throughout the day, whatever your mind now creates, you now enjoy the benefits of, raising your metabolism, as a lighter, thinner, unstoppable, healthier, this better you, burns food, fat, weight, and calories, more naturally, easier and better, than ever before.

You begin to enjoy plenty of life giving water washing you clean inside and out throughout the day, water, now a wonderful type of snack.

Less is more, you fill up sooner, your body is fulfilled, your mind is more calm and focused, finding serenity as well as inner and outer peace, smaller portions consumed off smaller plates, eating only at mealtimes in designated eating areas, free of media distractions, make you more self-aware of filling up sooner, being satisfied, and knowing when enough is enough.

Having put your foot down this time once and for all, you succeed here automatically and unbeatably, your automatic mind, and higher consciousness, working any and all of this out unbeatably in your favor completely, in ways both known and unknown to you.

Regular meals of healthy foods throughout the day, completely fulfill you, just a taste for small mouthful, later in the day, it's enough for you, you feel comfortable you are calm, you remain relaxed, slow and steady deep breathing, guides your way.

You begin to take better care of yourself choosing what's better for you to eat and choosing to enjoy and like any and all of this even better while rising above and forgoing childish instincts and habits, taking better care of yourself now was an adult.

Less is more, you fill up sooner, and it is really all right, or perhaps just OK to leave some of your meal on the plate, as you leave the table, this is really just fine with you.

Less is more, you fill up sooner, taking better care of yourself as an adult, your greatest reward now success and breakthrough, while remaining clear of kiddy foods, just a very small taste is enough, a small mouthful allows you to enjoy the taste, and the sensation is enough to satisfy you completely.

You begin to take better care of yourself choosing what's best for you to eat and choosing to enjoy and like any and all of this even better while rising above and forgoing childish instincts and habits, taking better care of yourself now was an adult.

You in this new and better chapter of your life now and forever always savor the time that you take to eat, just a small morsel of any food now more than satisfies any of your cravings, you now lighter, thinner, healthier and better.

You reward yourself by drinking plenty of cold water, washing you clean inside, you now certain and self-assured, a large more high protein breakfast takes better care of you throughout the entire day.

You relax and rather than attempting to control flow of life, a new and better way to live in this brand new chapter of your life, allowing natural perfection to take place around you free from your control, you appreciate life as you are now relaxing beyond former limits and barriers into a brand new place, feeling better about yourself, you are now unstoppable.

You find yourself relaxing your entire body, as well as your emotions, mind and spirit, resting better at night time, sleeping better through the night, calm and relaxed, at emotional peace, and should you need to consume anything in the middle of the night, the cold glass of water takes better care of you and will support you in newer better ways, lighter, thinner, healthier better, liberating a thinner you, more perfect there you are now, doing better than ever before.

I wonder if you yet realize how easy it is for you to become lighter, thinner, healthier and better, as you metabolism goes up, in ways most healthy and better for you, releasing and letting go of, 13, 18, 24, 26, even 29lbs., doing better for yourself while remaining true to you.

Seizing the unstoppable inspiration in this moment and empowering yourself, you release barriers from the past and flow ever onward, ever more certain and self-assured knowing all of this to be true.

You have moved into a brand new chapter of your life, re-tuned, recalibrated, reset, as you have now decided to release all discomfort and imbalance, forgive yourself and heal the situations from the past, releasing them, each and every breath and heartbeat the situations and emotions less important, while loving yourself better and more unconditionally instead.

In this brand new and better chapter of your life, you make better choices and decisions, your impulses, your actions and reactions, now working in your favor, in ways completely self-supportive.

You slow down while you eat, less is more, you fill up sooner on healthy foods, from smaller plates, you now more attracted to higher levels of protein and less carbohydrate.

Having grown up just a bit more in this brand new chapter of your life, while still able to have fun, you now realize that eating healthy is easy, you now loving yourself enough to take better care of yourself as good food tastes even better.

You begin to take on drinking plenty of life giving water washing you clean inside.

You begin to take the time and make the time to treat yourself better, bringing your exercise goals down to levels of ridiculous ease, for 30 seconds each time, two or three times a week, easily exceeding that time as you get into it better.

Walking, simply moving around more often, the joy and ease of movement, all become a second nature to you.

You begin to open up your mind and your life to new friendships and associations, perhaps even finding a workout buddy to work out with.

You begin to generate limitless amounts of self motivation and self discipline to get the job done

Your automatic and dynamic subconscious mind is working this out to maximum benefit in ways both known and unknown to you.

You begin to do things you now love that generate ultimate results.

I wonder if you even yet realize how easy it will be for you as it is now happening automatically all around you.

You more easily release your addiction to food, your dynamic mind now in ways both known and unknown to you, works out all issues, completely generating new and improved methods of habit and behavior which achieve results and more and more complete results.

It's almost as if someone from deep, deep inside of you has switch, a dial, thermostat of some kind, motivating and child-like new interest and excitement in your life.

You now mightier and more powerful than any challenges, mightier now and forever rising up to face down any and all, boredom or depression, cleverly adapting to all, rising up to meet and overwhelm all, the greater you are challenged, the better you are, while finding joy in greater movement.

The weight just seems to find new ways to melt it off and keep it off.

A newer and better loving heart guides your way into a better day and a better way.

Your clever and adaptive mind finds new and better ways to remain calm, focused, peaceful and serene, or simply clear.

Your automatic and dynamic mind is beginning to make permanent adjustments and prevailing improvements, in ways known and even unknown to you, which work thrivingly, while only, precisely in your favor, to balance, heal and restore all that you are.

Free forever you are and you remain of ever, ever eating without thinking again, feeling more powerful than ever.

This ever functioning mind of yours is almost like someone has from deep, deep inside of you, reset a switch, a dial, a thermostat, or a computer of some kind, that works in your favor, or perhaps, it's like a light coming down from on high all around you, that improves your eating habits dramatically.

Less is more, you fill up sooner, smaller dishes, smaller plates, smaller bowls, eating only at mealtimes, free of media distractions, actively and more enjoyable better body movement, which allows you to burn in surprisingly effective and automatically dynamic ways, food, fat, weight, calories, while consuming enjoyably plenty of water, washing you clean inside and out.

In this new and forever improve chapter of your life, you choose to eat breakfast, even a large breakfast, and a much lighter lunch, and even lighter dinner, feeling most wonderfully and very completely fulfilled, mentally, emotionally, even spiritually, most especially, feeling fulfilled physically.

Forever free of ever using food as a reward, you are and happily remain, as you are taking better care of yourself filling up much sooner, a small taste is enough for you.

Both now and forever gone are the days of overdoing it, taking your life in a greater and better stride, treating yourself as your own best friend, loving yourself like someone you care about, better movement now yours, as you now treat yourself like someone you care about, more emotionally clear, and goal determined to make this happen unbeatably.

You are free of the eating, overeating, thrivingly, of over-wanting food in anyway, feeling better and complete, having satisfied yourself and your needs, doing better for yourself in every way, most especially whenever you're feeling good or even if feeling lonely, depressed, bored, and when you have too much time on your hands; even if that seems to happen way too often.

Your eating times now become and remain about sustenance, sustaining your body, and taking better care of yourself, and this brand new chapter of your life, doing better for yourself, a small taste is enough, a small taste is satisfying enough for you.

Once you've tasted the flavor of sweets or fatty foods, you're done.

You eat smaller portions, filling up sooner, and feel satisfied about yourself, even more so about your life.

You eat more slowly and fill up sooner; all things once your weakness, now your greatest strength.

Smaller portions, smaller plates, smaller bowls, with smaller portions, eaten more slowly, whether it's ice cream, bread, or pasta, just a smaller taste, just a few bites, just enough for you, often even leaving some of each and every meal behind in the plate or bowl, has you doing better and a better for yourself, while with others or even alone, most especially in ways both known and unknown to you.

Almost as if you've grown up just a little bit more, things of the past now done and finished, you now better and better feeling fine, empowered.

You now know that you have in fact, have entered a brand new chapter of your life, a brand new age, a better place, taking better and better care of yourself as a part of this now more grown up to you, more focused and enabled, inspired, you find, take a pace, and enjoy the rhythm, of the time it takes, to prepare your meals and put yourself first, enthusiasm and energetic, to take better care of yourself while easily relaxing barrier free, putting your needs first.

When it comes to losing weight you start out and stay strong and focused, and continue as if driven on from high above, with great energy and drive; almost as if floating down a river, so even after losing 4, 9, 15, 21 pounds you seem to continue to float and flow ever onward to where you need to be, for ever released, healed and forgiven, forever free of any and all now and forever released and outgrown habits.

As a way of taking better, even best care of yourself, you find more joy in movement and moving around, finding reasons to move your body, and someday, even now, find that as you move around more you feel better becoming lighter, thinner, healthier, better, more energetic, doing anything and everything it takes to make this happen.

Finding excuses to move your body, even short walks, choosing to move, joy and movement, movement is joy, so enjoyable, in ways both known and unknown to you, you now so true and effective.

You are easily able to see, to notice and to remember, that you have and continue to improve your life, through, a better diet, proper for an adult, healthy for an adult, better for yourself, easily able to bring walking as a form of exercise into your life, a few times each week, bring the goal down to a level of ridiculous ease.

Each and every time that it's time to exercise, you recognize that a superior person just gets up and does it, exercise wise, so you do, you like it, you love it, it feels great, so very enjoyable, a special gift of longevity that you give yourself.

You are powerfully free of eating or wanting to eat or craving anything to eat just because food is around.

You are powerfully free of eating or wanting to eat or craving anything to eat just because you are or might be lonely, depressed, bored, and when you have too much time on your hands.

You eat when hungry, choosing to eat to live, forever free of eating when not hungry; all emotional issues you once had are now clearing, cleansing, evaporating, blown way and done.

You are powerfully free of eating or wanting to eat or craving anything to eat just because you are or might be emotionally distraught.

You are powerfully free of ever eating either during or when doing homework, for the greater the issue, the more focused, calmer and serene you remain inside, at inner peace, comfortable and more happy, the turn of the patient, hunger-free, lighter, healthier, thinner, better.

Whether alone or with other people, you choose to eat to live rather than living to eat.

You have entered a brand new chapter of your life doing better and better, your automatic mind is now working this out for you in ways most profound and effective, both known and unknown to you, in ways that release and heal, even forgive the past.

All of this leads to greater and more profound improvement in your life, both inside and out, better eating habits, regularly paced, with proper and more appropriate, more healthy, more nutritional, more appealing food for you, time to exercise, take better care of yourself, and love yourself better, all now a newer and better part of you, in this brand new chapter of your life.

Gone now and forever are the days of using food as a crutch to deal with stress or as a break or even as a reward.

When dealing with stress, your best possible choice is to take a break, have a glass of water, deep breathe, relax and calm down.

You choose to eat smaller portions of healthy food throughout the day, feeling so hunger-free and at home, complete and comfortable, all through the night, a glass of water, enough to calm down any and all hunger any time during the night, easily, affectingly, and as needed instantly.

All that you are, body, emotions, mind, even spirit, reset, re-tuned, recalibrated, unnecessary weight melts off, as a lighter, healthier, thinner and better you emerges.

More ready and enabled to love yourself, while releasing any and all imbalanced emotions, automatically, in ways known and unknown to you, more self loving and life supporting thoughts and feelings, guiding you into a place of higher and better nights in your life, learning to love all that you are, body, emotions, mind, even spirit, as all generates a peaceful soothing harmony, all around you, loving your body enough and yourself enough to break through and succeed here unbeatably.

Learning to enjoy movement and body activity, you move around more, all of this just seems to be, automatic, and effective, finding joy and more movement in your body and in your life.

You are powerfully free of eating or wanting to eat or craving anything to eat just because food is around.

You are powerfully free of eating or wanting to eat or craving anything to eat just because you are or might be stressed, most especially if challenged in any way, challenge-oriented problem-free forever .

You will only receive powerful and precise, highly effective beneficial improvement in the correct and most powerful ways from this, going into this wonderful relaxation state faster, deeper, stronger and better, with more limitless results in my unlimited ways every time you repeat this extremely enjoyable, wonderful, dynamic, highly effective and precise breakthrough exercise.

You more easily rise up now to meet any and all challenges, attacking the challenges, while making better choices and remaining peaceful and serene inside, your mind cleverly adapting breakthroughs here now in place known and unknown, to you.

When dealing with stress, your best possible choice is to take a break, have a glass of water, deep breathe, relax and calm down.

You choose to eat smaller portions of food throughout the day, feeling so hunger-free and at home, complete and comfortable, all through the night, a glass of water, enough to calm down any and all hunger any time during the night, easily, affectingly, and as needed instantly.

You truly find now in this brand new chapter of your life, protein is much more soothing and satisfying, keeping you hunger-free, the best possible choice rather than loading up on carbohydrates as once was done in now finished and over, past chapters of your life.

Whether at work or at home, you have chosen to rise above stress heroically, and to take things at a different pace with inner certainty, with the skill of a mighty master in your life, at work and at home, easily surmounting any and all challenges, problem-free challenge-oriented.

It is almost as if, your automatic mind is now focusing on areas of your body that need to be reduced, and that you will learn to love better, and see what's new and better.

Long before your first bite, the sight and the smell of the food begins to fill you up, you fill up sooner, maybe even four times faster, feeling satisfied, free of ever eating from stress, you choose to deep breathe, relax, and unwind, free again of ever dieting, you choose to restructure, anything and everything that creates new habits, actions, reactions, inspirations, desires, that automatically, in ways both known and unknown to you, automatically working themselves out, generating, a lighter, healthier, thinner, better, more energetic, more movement oriented you.

As it is time to let go of the weight of the past, so any and all additional extra weight from the past, is now released into the past, in ways both known and unknown to you, both physically, emotionally, mentally, and in every way.

The past now done and over, you know, you are both now and forever released and freed, lighter, healthier, thinner, better, more energetic, your mind now adaptably creating strategies, methods, solutions, hunger-free, fulfilled, happier, truly feeling protected by your life, all things, everything, every thought and feeling, healthier foods now more appealing, less is more, small tastes are enough, you fill up sooner, breaking through here unbeatably, unstoppable, lighter, healthier, thinner, better, higher metabolism, adaptably eating only when hungry.

In this brand new and better chapter of your life, you now, and forever, unstoppably move forward, unbeatably, you thrive and succeed, as slow and steady deep and relaxing breath guides your way, your stress simmers down, as you relax, more barrier free, more stress-free, you realize and recognize a new truth in your life, as serenity guides your way, into a lighter, more energetic, more enhanced, more balanced, better you.

Weight Extras 2

Knowing this now to be true, almost as if someone or something from deep, deep inside of you, has reset a switch, a dial, a thermostat, or a computer of some kind which is now working unstoppably in your favor, you relax a deeper now, calm you, restore you, empower and make you mighty, even heroic, and a new chapter of your life begins.

In this brand new and reset better chapter of your life, the gift of control is now yours, chewing and eating more slowly, and filling up sooner.

You eat to live, and food is less interesting, you fill up sooner, actually beginning to fill up along before the first bite, simply the smell of food from a distance, begins to fill you immediately.

In this brand new and better chapter of your life, new habits, creating health and freedom, generate a more exciting passion for life, a greater desire to drink water, less is more, you fill up sooner, eating places free of media distractions.

Small plates, dishes, bowls, more appropriate eating times, now about sustenance, which means sustaining your body, emotions, and mind, as you now more compassionately treat yourself like an adult, taking better care of you, as any and all no longer needed weight just seems to simply melt away.

Less hungry you are physically, emotionally, and mentally.

Finding inner peace, you now more satisfied by life, more peaceful, serene and steady especially should you ever feel hungry.

Relaxing beyond former barriers, those barriers now and forever melt away and are now gone forever.

In this brand new and better chapter of your life, struggle-free, you relax, and release stress and anxiety, almost as if someone from deep, deep inside of you, has reset a dial, switch, computer, or mechanism of some kind, allowing you to thrive and succeed here, re-identifed, forgiven, healing, whole, and released, lighter, thinner, better, calmer, with a higher metabolism, burning automatically food, fat, weight, and calories, any and all of this seems to be happening automatically, as if it has a mind of its own, as your automatic mind now generates this and makes it so.

For the greater the stress, the more the serene, and peaceful, your breathing becomes, more slow, more steady, more regular, all of this just seems to be happening, and so it is and it remains forever, working in your favor.

The greater the stress, the more steady your breath, the greater the stress and anxiety, the more calm you become.

In this brand new and better chapter of your life, you take better care of yourself as an adult should, taking all things in stride, making and taking the time to prepare good food and make healthy choices.

You now more easily bring your exercise goals down to levels of ridiculous, simple ease, taking ten to fifteen seconds a day, three times a week, to do something like move around or just take a walk, easily getting into the rhythm and sustaining it for a half hour to an hour; it's amazing how the time goes by so quickly and happily, enjoyably, feeling more fulfilled.

Smoking Cessation

Stop Smoking – Back on Track,
This Time Forever

The more you see another person smoking, the more smoke-free and cigarette-free you become, for any temptation by them or any of their actions, the stronger your resolve and life giving beneficial results, and the more free of their silly self-destructive habits, you become, almost as if seeing them smoke means absolutely and completely nothing at all to you at all, as a safer, healthy, stronger, more resolute, happier, more centered, more determined than ever [man/woman] gloriously rises up and emerges heroically forever.

Most especially if ever challenged again by the sight of your [husband / wife smoking], the smell of any cigarettes is unpleasant and perhaps annoying, reaffirming why you are a non smoker now.

Whether calm, comfortable, and feeling fulfilled, or even if you are at any time even in the slightest way feeling lonely and upset, you have truly and even more completely grown up and moved forward, more secure and resolute within your life to remain smoke-free, cigarette-free.

In this brand new chapter of your life, you've come to realize that you are far too important, for yourself and for your loved ones, most especially for yourself, to ever begin smoking again, finished now, in a new chapter of your life, clearly and absolutely free of cigarettes and smoking, forever.

Feeling great, better and more inspirational supportive feelings, making you feel better, all old stumbling blocks, now completely unimportant to you, dissolved, in the most important of ways.

Your correct response to any amount of any and all stress or anxiety, is to take slow and steady deep cleansing, refreshing breaths, while achieving an easily achieved yet profoundly powerful foundational state of soothing calm, centeredness and peacefulness, as this only grows stronger and better on each and every breath, allowing you to release and detach from stress around you, truly knowing and feeling this, while feeling an embracing, loving glow within your heart for the people you care about, most especially for yourself.

You now know as a true fact, you are too important to ever smoke anything ever again, and so it's done, feeling great.

Almost as if someone from deep, deep inside of you has reset a switch, a dial, a computer or a thermostat of some kind, easily allowing you to once and for all, completely and forever, to always and forever cherish remaining smoke-free cigarette-free, not because I say so, but because it's the nature of your own mind in ways both known and unknown to you, true, in the most effective and surprising, even clever and surprising brilliantly adaptive ways, achieving breakthrough ultimate success here.

Your days of shame and embarrassment over, feeling free at long last, you relish the joy and the pride of being a smoke-free cigarette-free [man/woman.]

Whatever once stood in your way, in previous and now done finished chapters of your life, you now have risen up, become mightier than, stepped forward from and beyond and over from, and are now free of that old stuff, simply unimportant - now you are important, just doing better and better, free at long last, truly feeling and knowing greater and greater levels of magnificence and success.

Happy and clear as to why you have quit smoking, you have regained your life, what a gift, what a relief!

You now any challenge to your health, your mind and your spirit are the greatest of healers, functioning fully and precise yet adaptive measure to achieve unbeatable success, you know this is leading a healthier life.

So happy and relaxed, to be forever free of any smoking addiction in every way, now smoke-free, cigarette-free, feeling a glow of liberation, safety, support, improving health, and you know this to be true, as your body and mind knitting you back together again, your mind and your spirit the most powerful of healers, your mind easily achieving any all of this, every thought, every feeling, every action, every reaction, leading you to greater and more dynamic and increasing levels of success.

This is now you and your life, always and forever, always getting stronger and better, more clear and resolute, than ever before, on each and every breath, on each and every heartbeat, every blink of your eyes, while you're awake, while you are asleep, while you are having comfortable and happy support of pleasant dreams, freedom yours now, there and here now, breaking through thus unbeatably.

Smoking Extras

Whenever you take a breath, you are more and more smoke free, cigarette free.

You now have forever given up smoking to gain back your life. You quit smoking as if your life depended on this, and so it does, and so it is, so you have, so you've done it, and so that is now and forever done. You succeed, almost like it has and will be for 50 years, you feel great.

You are and now remain, smoke-free, cigarette-free, while now and forever within a brand new chapter of your life, forever free of ever using smoking and cigarettes as a pacifier, almost as if someone from deep, deep inside of you has reset a switch, a dial, or a thermostat of some kind which is now activated from the deepest places inside of you most meaningful to you, and ability that has allowed you to reset, recalibrate, and rebalance yourself, truly knowing forever that you have moved on, unbeatably, into a brand new chapter of your life, smoke-free and cigarette-free, now and forever, even finding clever reasons and excuses to remain that way.

You are doing wonderfully well, I wonder if you even yet realize how truly easy this is for you, both now and forever.

Forgiving and releasing the past you are empowered, you are liberating your mighty inner hero, you are releasing, healed, forgiven, and loving yourself better, in a brand new and better chapter of your life, now, so much easier, so much better, than ever before, smoke free, cigarette free.

You are and you forever remain smoke free, cigarette free, most especially while at work for the day and thinking, finding mental clarity, focus, a shopper and crisper understanding, with better insights, memory, and recall, feeling better about yourself and how great you feel, smoke-free, cigarette-free.

Most especially whenever you are in the bathroom, think about heading into a bathroom, think about using the bathroom in any way, any thought of a bathroom now becomes place of power, transformation, triggering feelings, thoughts, actions, and reactions, that will keep you smoke free cigarette-free in the each and every moment, in fact, you begin to realize that cigarettes have no place in your life, and most especially no place in the bathroom, so both now and forever your smoke-free cigarette-free, feeling wonderful about yourself and your life.

Barrier free you are, you become and you are and now so completely motivated and inspired, you forever now remain.

You know, in fact, it's almost as if Divinely inspired just getting into your well-deserved, much inspired and appreciated success and freedom here, almost as if someone from deep, deep inside of you, has reset a switch, a dial, a thermostat, or computer of some kind, safely and forever liberating you from smoking and from cigarettes forever.

Breathing easier clean air, your life now more fulfilling, total, and complete, now, this brighter, better, chapter of your life is now yours and has unbeatably begun.

Remaining forever and completely true to yourself now in this new chapter of your life unbeatably, happier, healthier and freer, having once and for all, forever put your foot down, as you are and you remain forever, smoke free cigarette free, most especially whenever you are with your spouse/husband/wife is smoking or is relating to smoking in any way whatsoever;.

Truly you now, a shining example to him/her, showing him/her, inspiring him/her, to a brighter, better, path to a healthier, happier life, extended life, more determined than ever before.

For the more you see him/her smoking, the obstinate and determined you are to stay and forever remain, smoke free, cigarette free, the harder anyone tries to draw you back in, the more smoke fee and healthier you stay and become, completely contrary to smoking anything and everything you remain and become.

The more you see someone else smoke, the greater and more unstoppable your urge becomes to forever remain smoke-free cigarette-free.

Life giving water washing you clean inside, keeping you forever and better more enjoyably smoke-free, cigarette-free.

The more challenged you become by seeing or smelling another person smoking, the more obstinate you completely become to forever remain, the opposite of them, in other words, you, completely reconditioned, to become and forever remain, smoke-free cigarette-free.

You are now and you cleverly remain smoke-free, cigarette-free, most especially in the morning, feeling better and more rejuvenated in the morning, smoke-free, cigarette-free, your new and even better way to kick start your even better day, always feeling better having made a healthier and correct choice, so much more now easily focused and stuck with unbeatably, adaptively and cleverly, having relaxed beyond former limits and barriers into the very best chapter of your life, smoke-free cigarette-free.

As a function of this brand new and better chapter of your life, you revolutionize your life and your world, doing anything and everything, to be effective while staying true to a new and improved smoke-free, cigarette-free you.

I wonder if you even yet realize how easy is going to be to remain smoke-free, cigarette-free as you walk from place to place, finding better ways to take care of yourself, and keeping your mind focused on more important things, like staying healthy, enjoying yourself, and being more prosperous, whenever walking, smoke-free cigarette-free.

The love that you have in your heart for your spouse, in all of your very best moments together, and the love you have for your family, coupled with your ability to become a shining example of the smoke-free, cigarette-free life, all combined together in harmony to break you through here unbeatably.

With each and every breath and heartbeat, you now doing so much better, succeeding brilliantly, supported by every past victory, triumph, breakthrough, and success, you've ever had.

Your lungs begin to clear as you deep breathe and relax, your breath expanding, as your lungs open, with each and every breath your stress begins to evaporate and disappear, for the greater the stress, the more soothing and regular your breath, the more serene and peaceful you are and you become, or just otherwise remain.

The greater the stress, whether it's family time, social situations, or any conversation, allows you to heroically rise up and become a mighty nonsmoker.

You are and you now and forever remain smoke, free cigarette free, most especially when you are downstairs feeding the puppies. You enjoy your dog's company and playfulness so much better, so much more loyal and true, so much more loving, playful and fun, smoke-free cigarette-free.

You are and you forever remain smoke-free cigarette-free, while taking a shower, taking much better care of yourself, as you luxuriate in the relaxing waters remaining clear, cleaner, healthy, better in body, emotions, mind, and spirit, as a new and brighter healing harmony now embraces you, you can practically even feel it.

You are and you now and forever remain smoke, free cigarette free, most especially before you go in to work.

You are and you now and forever remain smoke, free cigarette free, most especially going into buildings or if when you are coming out of building or near the exit to work.

You are and you shall forever remain clear and free of ever craving any sort of cigarette or anything to smoke, benefiting every thought, feeling, energy or whether it's at 9:50 AM, 9:55 AM, 10:00 AM, 10:05 AM, most especially, 10:10 AM.

You look forward to the smoke-free, cigarette-free, easier breathing better life, your clever and wise Unstoppable determined mind is set.

Right now, right here, this is your brand new dawning day of freedom.... free forever of any inhalers, easier and better breathing and longevity and greater healing and with your breathing becoming healthier, return to healthy, and normal, plenty of air and breath for you to go around in your life smiling, happy, confident, polished, shiny, new, renewed, better than ever before, all disharmony and imbalance draining away, harmony and balance, light and healing guide your way.

Ahhhhh, it feels so great to be so nicotine free.

You are now and forever remain smoke-free, cigarette-free, most especially if any time whenever you are or might be feeling emotional, as a feeling is just a feeling, a thought just a thought, so no matter how lightly or strongly stressed, angry, excited, or any emotion you experience, you are cleverly and adaptably determined to become stronger and better at being smoke-free, cigarette-free.

You more easily and readily welcome and feel more and more at home in any place that is a smoke free environment, being safe, feeling calm and serene, more and more smoke free, cigarette free, before, during and after, walking into any store/appointment, or any place that is smoke free cigarette free, just like you are, as your energies have upgraded, smoking has lifted off you and you are lighter and freer than ever before.

For the greater the challenge, or the greater the stress, or maybe the greater the potential for you worrying about those you love in any situation, the mightier and more smoke-free, cigarette-free you become and forever remain, inspired, empowered, and able, even enabled, to recognize and fully commit to the idea, the foundationally life improving and life extending, correct and only choice idea, that you have once and for all you have put your foot down, and made a permanent life improving decision, loving yourself enough to have things work in your favor, this time you the unstoppable winner forever, smoke-free, cigarette-free.

The unconditional love and support you have for others now translates into love you have to yourself and as a mighty and unstoppable, forever part of this extended love for yourself, growing ever stronger and more powerful, is to give yourself a smoke-free cigarette-free life, and to happily extend your life, love, wisdom and guidance to be there for those that you love so much.

And so there it is, and there you now and forever remain, you now and forever whole-heartily enjoy a hot cup of coffee while cleverly and adaptably, most effectively, choosing to remain smoke-free, cigarette free after dinner, finding pleasure and happiness, a complete and total winner in your life, and a master of our world, smoke-free cigarette-free most especially after any meal.

You choose to love rather than to worry, to be concerned, and direct your actions into safe, sane while even channeling the wisdom and guidance you now know you have, to assist those you love in your life, also more easily able to skill and wisdom of the master, to use all of your very best intentions, wisdom, insights, talent, skills, inspirations, intuition, to become and forever remain smoke-free, cigarette-free.

Your clever and adaptive automatic subconscious mind is now easily, skillfully, adaptably, and forever working out anything and everything it takes, marvelously effective ways, both known and unknown to you, to generate and easily create a smoke-free, cigarette-free life, breathing easier, loving yourself enough to stay this way, promoting and generating anything and everything it takes to stay this way, with a lighter more determined, more heroic and upbeat attitude.

You are and you remain smoke-free, cigarette-free, inventing new, better, clever, and even adaptive and fulfilling ways, to stay that way, most especially in the morning, struggle-free, and easy, so effective, most especially 30 minutes after waking up and easily reinforced for during and after, a light snack.

Your body comes in to a better alignment and a better place, digestion and elimination systems, and better harmony, better lubrication, now so much better and effective smoke-free, cigarette-free, digestion and elimination working better having faster, easier and more frequent bowl movements.

You are and you remain, smoke-free, cigarette-free, any time food is around, most especially after having a meal.

In any situation that is emotional, you are more easily able to be successful, rising above any and all challenges, smoke-free cigarette-free, bound and determined to stay that way, most especially if you are or may be upset, stressed or excited emotionally.

For the greater the challenge once was to stay smoke-free cigarette-free, the more easily unchallenged you are and you are unstoppably able to remain this way now and forever.

You are easily generating inspirational empowerment, so effective, motivated from every past victory, triumph, breakthrough, inspirational success, and all moments in your life when you were unbeatable, to stay free of smoking and cigarettes, smoke-free, cigarette-free, craving free, comfortable in your own skin, in any and all situations, absolutely determined, like a masterful hero of legend, all of your focus and will, smoke-free cigarette-free, not because I say so, but because it is in fact natural for a mind to do this, and so it remains forever, most a specially at a movie, taking a flight, in an airport, during a class, meeting with friends, anytime, you remain a shining example of the smoke-free cigarette-free life.

Your skillful and adaptive subconscious automatic mind now works to start for you, in amazingly successful ways, you remain in a brand new chapter of your life, all things in the past chapters of your life that once caused you to smoke, now smoke-free cigarette-free, your greatest urge to remain and stay that way, rising above past challenges, you free and safe, treating yourself properly, knowing you should, so to now you forever do.

Personal Development

Generating Prosperity, Trust In Life, and Health

You are now truly and profoundly relaxed, feeling great. You are now ready and completely open to new and more expanded possibilities and the inspiration of improving your life, as all of you, your body, your emotions, your mind and even spirit are activated powerfully, profoundly, effectively and adaptively, in the most unstoppable of ways, both now and forever dynamically working in your favor, taking any and all necessary strides and steps while making beneficial moves, trusting in your higher guidance and instincts, while well deservedly you, becoming totally healed, abundant and even rich.

You are placing your order with the supreme higher power to get want you need. As you relax, you are relaxing deeper and further, further and deeper on each and every breath, and on each and every heartbeat.

Just as if resetting a switch, a dial, a thermostat, or even activating your powerful life redirecting computer of some kind, from deep, deep within, deep, deep inside of you, you are now being perfectly guided to activate only your very best, easily attracting only the very best, truly repelling all of the rest, activating both release and forgiveness, while completely releasing any and all past blockages, all of those dissolving, while activating self- generating, levels of ever increasing happiness, and generating your ability to stay centered and focused, to rise above, truly feeling centered, serene, peaceful, totally relaxed and stress-free.

More and more profoundly relaxed, easily feeling yourself so rested, it's *almost as if* you've had *a nine hour nap and a seven hour full body massage, back and feet and legs feeling marvelous,* feeling wonderful, as any and all old blockages as any and all stress seems to be melting far, far away from your body, emotions, mind, and even spirit, as a new and ever-present harmony and ability to transcend any and all past limits from previous chapters of your life, is now bubbling up from both heart and mind, in *eternal profound harmony,* generating, a centered peacefulness, that as in previous chapters of your life, you've simply dreamed about, yet now, is all around you, as if the energy is flowing from your body, all around you reinforcing any and all of this, as you are both strengthened and rejuvenated, as you now feel wonderful.

All of these recalibrations, actually feel like and seem to be, strengthening your immune system so that your skin and hair remain healthy, your aches in pains are easily becoming alleviated, dissolved, and dynamically controlled by the fortified, mighty power that is you.

Open to better right now, you are receiving the good in your life, only thinking and imagining in more positive, more and more self-supporting terms, while creating an ability to transcend any and all limits, all the time, as each and every day, it's becoming easier and more perfect for you, so precise and so dynamically effective. This new abundant energy and abundant you, easily, readily and dynamically, is generating the kind of energy that allows you to magnetically attract a wonderful caring successful wealthy man / woman.

At bedtime, you are skillfully allowing your mind to put the day and its past events, as well as the day tomorrow shall be and its future events, up on a shelf, so you can rest peacefully, right through the night. From deep, deep inside, you truly know, yesterday has taken care of you, and tomorrow will do just the same. All of your yesterdays have allowed you to learn or succeed, failure-free, and all of your tomorrows will be just the same.

So at bedtime, each and every night, you simply put your day on a shelf, put your head upon your pillow, finding relaxation and comfort as your muscles comfortably unwind, melt away, relax, you close your eyes and simply go to *sleep!* Just as you've done so many other nights in the past, sleeping peacefully right through the night, easily able to fall back to sleep, whenever you need to, you are just doing better and better.

As these powerful forces that direct your life on now being re-calibrated on each and every breath, and each and every heartbeat, you are redefining yourself beyond any and all past limits, to allow yourself to thrive here becoming a mighty magnet for prosperity, whether known or unknown to you.

You are cleverly and masterfully releasing both blockages and restrictions, fluidly and adaptively, in ways that only work very best for you. So smooth, so seamless and so effectively, finding and liberating prosperity into your life all around you, as you become a mighty magnet for prosperity, and better finance, so very easily inspired as your mind is working on improving all aspects of your life, while you were awake, while you were asleep and even while you dream, peacefully sleeping through the night, feeling relaxed, so refreshed, and so very rejuvenated.

From now on, each and every morning, joyously awakening, you are ready to seize the day, and make it your very own, as you are doing better and better, in each and every way, feeling lighter, more energetic, and more unstoppably inspired. You are and you dynamically remain more easily able to visualize and feel your success and your business prospering. You command it to come now, from heart and mind, and the part of you which is Divine, generates it all around you.

You are so easily able to be just the *right weight*, feeling good about yourself, loving yourself, caring about yourself, taking care of yourself. So when you go eat, you will enjoy it and do it peacefully, caringly and lovingly while remaining forever free of rushing because now it's about you and your good, ever improving, sweet life.

You are and you remain grateful to be blessed with health, happiness, growing wealth, creativity, success, while guiding good family, children and people. As you are loved and favored. Ask now and know you shall receive.
From deep down inside, from all that you are right now and are growing into, fulfilling yourself into, you truly know you are richly blessed now and forever, trusting in all that

is, and remains, and evolves into, the rest of your life while generating only the very best.

You come to trust and now all of this to be true and each and every day and night, while upon each and every breath, each and every heartbeat, all of this is becoming easier and better as you recognize this truly from places deep inside of you.

Becoming a Healer and Activating Inner Strength

You have determined within your mind and within your soul, in fact truly throughout all that you are, in fact all of you, body, emotions, mind, and spirit, in Divine harmony and blessing, that *you are mightier than any challenge that will arrive in your life*, as you are the one who is both magnetizing and repelling any and all challenges that arrive or might arise within your life.

You trust in the true fact, the very true fact, a foundational truth of your life, that you are powerfully and universally protected, and will stay safe, secure, and strong, for the greater the challenge, the mightier your trust.

For beyond belief there is faith, beyond faith, there is knowing, you now knowing right now in this moment of deep and soothing relaxation and effectively inspired realization, you simply and truly know, that you are mightier and more creatively adaptive than any challenge, that may or may not arise in your life, because you are now the mighty one in your life, and in this moment, you are feeling as if you are entering a brand new chapter of your life, rising above any and all challenges, both real and imagined, and the most truly and powerful and highly effective of ways.

For the greater your perceived challenge or vulnerability, the greater and more adaptively effective your strength. For the mightier the shadow, the greater your shadow vanquishing light. You choose to only experience what you can handle, just as always, effectively handling it all.

And now powerfully you rely on the fact that you are mightier than any challenge that may ever arise in your life, and just as sure as the sun always comes up in the morning, your light shines from your heart and your mind in powerful focus, healing determination, and the ability to rise above, vanquishing any and all challenges as needed, because you now see yourself in a brand new chapter of your life, heroic and protected, you now the mighty one.

Whatever you experience, you now completely unstoppable and all that you wish to accomplish and in fact will and do accomplish, you effectively accomplish, either mightily or fearlessly. For it has been said, *fear is like an empty vessel with a hole in it, it does nothing, it holds nothing, it is useless.*

In this brand new chapter of your life, you choose to simply rise above any and all challenges that you once found standing in your way into old and now forever done previous chapters of your life, shining the eternal light of heart and mind into places where the shadows may have once ever existed, removing uselessness from your life.

By relaxing, releasing, and letting go, you are allowing all the adversity to flow around you, and far, far away from you, what you are feeling, is more easily wonderful inside and out, rising to the very top, and becoming mighty once and for all. And you a feeling confident and inspired by your new and correct instantaneous reaction to this.

For in this new chapter of your life, the veil is lifted, it is done, it is blown away in the wind, far, far, far away from you, and with every heartbeat and breath you truly know better and deeper, truly better than any time in your life or past existence. You are bound and determined, even completely unstoppable, in moving forward in your life right now, free to do any work or challenge set out before you, magnetizing any and all challenges, for the greater the challenge, the mighty are more capable, the more powerful, more heroically determined and focused you are, in laser-beam like precision to breakthrough here, smiling at your successful outcome. You now determined to rise above it all, and forever always so it is.

In this brand new chapter of your life you are unstoppably forever free, you are free and moving forward, and like a mighty river running down the side of the mountain in the springtime, you flow over, around, beyond, through, and ever onward, to the places you best need to be. Just like a boulder in that fast running stream of water, you are polished by any and all previous experiences and past moments in your life, moving into the very best, as you are shiny and bright, seasoned, and better than ever before, evolving forward in your life.

With each and every heartbeat, and on each and every breath, each and every time you shake your head yes, in any conversation, you are more certain and sure, you are now and forever unblocked, fearless and dynamic, *free of embarrassment,* wide open as needed and when necessary psychically and psychically healed, activating your very best abilities in the most dynamic of ways, liberating the very best that you can be, and all that you are.

Your mighty inner hero and healer now active from deep, deep within yourself, is now one forever liberated. The part of you that is capable of saving children from great danger like fire is now working in your favor, to redirect against itself any challenges, negativity and shadowy energies that once ever stood in your way. For the greater that force, the more directed against itself becomes and the more free, shiny, and new you become, forever liberated, safe, and strong.

Feeling so relaxed right now, you are recalibrated, you are reset, you are rejuvenated, you are restarted, better than ever, you are shiny and new, a brand new and forever unstoppable, brand new beginning here for you, a gift from on high, as if starting out anew.

Your strongest, most important, most potent emotions, make you feel as though you are gaining strength, from any and all challenges that ever once stood in your way, for beyond belief you simply now just know that you are thriving and mighty in this ever growing stronger moment, stress-free, fearless, strong, healthy, whole, relaxed, with a higher metabolism, feeling safe, doing what's right and mighty for yourself and others while remaining adaptive and strong, for your inner wisdom and inner and outer light vanquishes all shadows. As you move beyond duality into glowing truth of oneness, it is obvious to all, most especially you, that you are flowing into a place of unity, strength and oneness.

As your vibration now rises, you are now feeling in a more potent place of health, healing, better life experience, strength, and heroic determination to get the job done, and so it is, and you now forever onward, into the very best moments of your life, as you are and you remain thriving and succeeding from deep, deep within, into the very best places that you can be, liberated, safe, strong, more dynamic than any challenge.

For in the past, any and all challenges which ever presented themselves to you have been an opportunity for powerful breakthroughs and success. You now have truly learned to see your life as a place of being failure free, choosing to either learn or succeed. Failure as limiting concept, now far away from you, drifting far away from your mind, your thoughts, habits and sense of feeling, your sense of being. You seize any and all opportunities to thrive and succeed moving forward, doing all things you set out to do honestly and serving you and all of those around you in the ways that best serve you all, in Divine oneness and balance.

You are rising above all challenges to a place of unity, free of limitation, liberating, unleashing feelings of unlimited success from deep, deep inside of you. Free of struggling and trying, you simply flow forward and are. Your heart and mind now in unstoppable balance, Divine love, light and healing, restoring you, while you are awake, while you are asleep, most especially while you sleep and dream, in serenity, happily, peacefully through the night, waking up each morning, ready to take on the day, even the night, rising above any and all challenges now as you are rejuvenated, heroic, and mighty, now an unstoppable force, of healing, light, enjoying and making the most of your life and all that you do, all that you are, all that you are to be, not because I say so, because this is in fact this is the truth.

And now true, you now know this, from your heart and mind now in powerful calm and determined focus, now in unstoppable harmony, now in powerful driving forward balance, creating and liberating the most important and potent moments of your life, and future. You now Divinely driven forward, into the very best chapters and experiences you can manifest, because you are now an unstoppable force in all that you are, all that you do, and all that you are to be, on each and every heartbeat, each and every breath, you now unstoppable, driven, and mighty and so it is.

Any and all of this creatively adapting itself to you, and your personality, habits. Life livelihood, and lifestyle, on each and every heartbeat and breath, every and any moment you blink your eyes and any conversation, you are becoming more self confident, centered, strong, even mighty, relaxing beyond all barriers, in greater health, exuberant, even prosperous.

Your correct and natural reaction to barriers as they arise, becoming more powerful as you are to be, most especially every time you repeat this enjoyable exercise and adaptively flexible and effective technique on your own, you are in fact healing an additional fifteen to eighteen years and stepping forward seizing all moments as opportunities as you break through unbeatably and undeniably into the very best moments of your life.

Your dynamic and mighty inner healer, now correctly and abundantly focused upon breaking through you here and adaptively healing you, you know right now healing, whole and healthy, getting only better and better, all is working in your favor as you are now dynamic and mighty, free at long last and it feels wonderful to be so free.

Success Motivation for Entrepreneurs/Business Professionals

Relax, float, drift, and dream, and as you do allow your mind in your magic nation to wonder, as if turning pages forward in a book, or fast forwarding on a DVD, to a time at some point in the future and ten, twelve, fifteen years down the road, you have achieved your success - you see yourself at that time living the dream you once envisioned, a successful, more motivated, more focused you.

Easily rising above any and all challenges, as you are thriving, succeeding, and moving forward, into better days, and a more supportive place in your life, each and every day, this future you thrives and succeeds, cleverly adapts, is adept and skillful, is more seasoned, more easily able to turn any challenges that might ever be facing defeat, into moments of glowing victory, snatching victory from the jaws of defeat, victory, triumph and breakthrough, that you make your own.

This future you, is making the kind of money you deserve, living in the kind of environment and home, surrounded by supportive, loving and nurturing family and friends, feeling well supported, cared for, and is taken care of, most especially by others, but even more especially, by yourself.

In your imagination now, allow the you that you are in this moment, to become one with the image in our mind, and to merge with, and become this future you right now, and feel a joining, a oneness, a commonality, that both you and he share, across time.

In these moments, you now growing more bold, more blockage-free, more wide open, more filled with happy and excited anticipation, ready to take on any of all events, circumstances, and challenges. In your imagination, imagine yourself now feeling inspired by professionals who have gone before you, for what they know, you know, for how they succeed, you succeed, for what they do, you do, for how they are inspired, you are inspired.

How they are free of mental blocks, most especially when dealing with excessive paperwork or contracts, so too are you, free at long last, feeling rejuvenated, reconditioned, foundationally recalibrated, and easily able to face down any and all challenges, easily able to rise up in order to get any job done, redefined and adaptive, driven and inspired, completely unbeatable, for the mightier the challenge, the more dynamic and inspired you are, driven forward to success unbeatably, mightier than any challenge presented.

Putting in the time you need to be better organized so that you are now in an unbeatably inspired and successful chapter of your life which begins right now and always remains, where you are and you remain, unbeatably and adaptively, creatively, better prepared, precise and efficient, absolutely willing to thrive and succeed, bold and mighty, unbeatably willing to do anything that it honestly takes to breakthrough here and succeed.

While you relax, your clever and adaptively creative subconscious automatic mind, is working up inspirational patterns of guidance, thoughts, actions, plans, and reactions, skillfully and cleverly adaptive, to once and for all allow you to always find reasons and even excuses, thoughts and feelings, driven to better inspirations to keep you permanently unblocked mentally.

As a professional, you now recognize, the greater the challenge, the more focused and directed your strength in proper proportion, seizing the moment of opportunity, activating your internal ability to become and always remain an excellent problem solver, in fact problem-free, challenge-oriented, for the greater the challenge, the more dynamic and effective you become, not because I say so, but because it's the nature of her own mind to do this unbeatably, and forever and always, so it is, so you remain, and so it gets done.

For you now, greater redefined, and recalibrated, unlimited, driven and determined for yourself and those you love, more easily able to become in a moment whenever faced by a challenge, to prevail through any and all challenges that might come up and not only expecting a positive outcome, but doing all that it takes both personally and professionally, to generate winning results, in unbeatable and professional form.

For the greater the challenge, the more mighty you become, and proactive you are in generating your success, almost as if embraced by the energy of every past victory, triumph, breakthrough, and success, that you've ever had, or for that matter, any one else has ever had.

Just like walking, or driving a car, riding a bicycle, or swimming, you are focused on the moves and the motion, free of ever second guessing and over-analyzing.

You know and trust your first instinct and impression, recalling, remembering, and performing, with the skill of a professional, for beyond belief, there is faith, beyond faith, there is knowing, and you know who you are, you trust in your instincts, you allow the harmony of heart and mind, to work together, generating inner wisdom, in your favor, to the mutual benefit of all around you, most especially yourself.

Redefined now you are and you remain in your mind, through these ten, or twelve, or fifteen years, or even more, worth of healing and well-seasoned inspired experience, liberating your inner mover and shaker.

Reinvented as well as being re-excited about your life and your work, you maintain high levels of excitement and inspiration. While remaining, clever, bold, dynamic, audacious, creative, easily navigating, even eager and driven as never before, following through up on any and all leads, and opportunities, to unbeatable levels of inspirational success.

By relaxing beyond the limits and barriers from now done and finished, over, previous chapters of your life, you now coalesce, most especially whenever speaking, getting any and all of your points across, concisely, sharply, well prepared, willing to do background research when needed, gaining all the facts and cohesively explaining them, at any and all times, most especially whenever when dealing with prospects and professionals.

In fact, feeling this to the level of knowing-ness right now, you now speaking so well, everything flowing, automatically, knowing when to speak, when to listen, when to remain silent, for all of these years of experience, relaxing and allowing it all to just come together in flow, feeling so inspired and so successful, so driven, each No puts you one step closer toward a Yes, no means explain it better to me, get me to understand so I can say yes.

You are feeling, almost as if someone has reset a switch, a dial, a thermostat, or a valve of some kind, even a computer of some sort, which is driving you forward unbeatably, completely reconditioned, recalibrated, rejuvenated, more proficient, activating greater wisdom for more experience, and from each and every experience.

You are more safe, more certain, more bold, more dynamic, more able, more serene, then at any other time before in your life, to break through right here, right now, unbeatably, as your inner wisdom glows in the harmony of heart and mind, as you are now caressed and embraced by the energy of success all around you, and for whatever that means, in ways both known and yet unknown to you, you now one with your success, thriving and succeeding unbeatably, living in these moments because they are now forever real and true, adaptive and more adjusted, more skillful, and more guided by higher wisdom, than ever before, you now an unbeatable success.

Public Speaking – Corporate Presentations

You always knew that your days as a public speaker would balance, improve, as you thrive. Right now is that point of power, making you completely unstoppable.

You are living and now thriving in a brand new chapter of your life, more barrier free than ever before.

Your correct response to anything challenging is to relax and flow, while from your heart and your mind and the harmony they embrace, it is as if you have reset a switch, a dial, a thermostat of some kind, or activated a powerful computer from deep within, in ways both known and unknown to you, to break you through here heroically.

Your breathing slows down, your heart rate slows down, and the words just seem to come and flow as if happening automatically all around you.

You now relax as you realize, any audience you speak to is an audience filled with supporters, and like little children being read a story, they want and need to hear what you have to say.

Any and all now and more forever done stress and nervousness, is now being alleviated from you and your life, as from your wise mind.

You are now forgiving, completely forgiving, healing, absolutely healing and releasing, any and all stressful blockages from the past that ever once stood in your way.

As you relax now, you rise up and become mighty, so heroically transcending any and all now for ever done and released, healed and forgiven limits, either real or imagined, known or unknown to you, and like a hero saving children from great danger like a fire, you thrive ever onward.

You have now chosen to rise above any and all challenges to forever and always become mighty in the face of adversity, and so it is and forever remains.

You allow yourself now powerfully to relax and flow, as the words come on their own, free of ever over-listening to what you are saying nor second-guessing yourself.

You are feeling a new and better sense of power, and you're simply one with the experience, one with the moment, flowing with the moment, teaching and presenting, forgiving and releasing disharmonious moments, and creating harmony in their place.

For now you know who you are, a mighty force of presentation, change, education, and healing in your life and in your world, and as well in anyone else's world, who comes into contact with you now and forever.

Anyone listening to what you have to say is cheering you on and supporting you. You are amongst friends, your greatest, most nurturing fans.

Your thoughts are the ones that matter.

Your sense of confidence, unbounded, as your automatic mind, wisely thrives and bathes in the knowledge that you are simply getting better and better, activating your greatest abilities while speaking, all peers or superiors, are now supporters and friends, the change taking place within you, generates a better day and a better moment in your life.

You relax, you articulate, and decide that this is play. The audience hears you, and appreciates you, as you generate self-love, as this becomes more like a party, and a fun experience, as you are free of ever being challenged by this experience in any way.

Should it become a challenge ever again, your mighty inner, wise hero will rise up, deal with this, and present in a relaxed way, as you are now teaching, a superior teacher, someone who illuminates and elucidates.

Any and all uncomfortable moments in the past, now so easily forgiven, healed and released.

Aahhhh, it feels so good to be so free once and for all, the burden has been released, you have stepped forward, your heart and mind glow, you smile inwardly, feel so great, to be so free forever.

Imagine relaxing ever deeper and even now, and imagine yourself immersed in an energy field located over your heart, now opening, and connecting to the golden-white light of the sun, as that sunlight now begins to fill your body, vanquishing any and all shadows and filling those areas with abundant golden-white light, releasing and all discomfort.

Returning comfort, ease, joy, inspiration, self-confidence, in abundant flow and supply, unconditional love for yourself, while your now innate and easily accessed abilities to teach, guide, impart knowledge.

It's truly amazing how much easier this is becoming for you, you now so relaxed in your own skin, in your own life, anytime in front of an audience, in person, over the phone, whether it's your computer or some other means, just imagine as you now come to know, how enjoyable experience for you this is and will remain forever as it is and will be.

You even begin to activate your mind to speak extemporaneously, relaxed enough to understand the lay of the land, the landscape which you are presenting, easily and more easily able to reason-out any and all things.

The greater the challenge, the mightier and more heroic you are, as you know this from places deepest and truest inside of you.

Your heart rate and breathing so relaxed and self-supporting, your skin temperature just right, all things working in tandem and in harmony, so effectively and surprisingly well, you either thrive and succeed, the choice is yours.

You begin to relax deeper and further, realizing that you have relaxed beyond formal limits and barriers into a brand new chapter of your life.

As you relax deeper and further, beyond words and their meaning, simply to a level of feeling and understanding, your full appreciation of the word relaxation and what it means, all that it means, you begin to physically memorize and are completely able to shift your energy to a place of calmness now, more easily than ever before, and at will as needed, most especially whenever challenged in your life.

Whether in calm or stressful situations, or especially whenever having to speak in front of any group. your mind automatically and forever shifts into a pattern of slow, soothing, deep, relaxation breath, empowering and inspiring you.

Each and every time you repeat this wonderfully enjoyable, ever more effective, self-perpetuating to success exercise on your own, so very enjoyable, you relax into this deeper, quicker, better, and easier, with even more startling, astonishing, and amazing confident success brimming with your very best attributes, from places known and unknown, most potent, powerful, and precise, from the deepest inside who you are, radiating out into the world all around you.

In every sense, your victorious mind, the resiliency of your spirit, beyond your consciousness, is now working out in the most highly effective in precise detail, methods, moves, strategies, abilities, talents, through release, forgiveness, and all the self-loving confidence, self-supporting, and inspirational necessary to break through here unbeatably in ways both known and unknown to you.

Public Speaking - for School Teachers

Your inner teacher now rising to surface, bubbling up to the top, focused and direct, having relaxed beyond any and all old and now done former barriers, into a brand new more motivated and confident chapter of your life, knowing what you have to share is crucial, critical, and important, enlightening, well received, as those who you are imparting knowledge to, are thirsty for what it is you have to share.

You become anew, remaining free of ever listening to what you were saying, your words are an extension of the thoughts, images, inspirations, and all that is within your mind, all speech just seems to flow, even free of second guessing yourself ever, feeling so confident and able, reconditioned, rejuvenated.

You relax, so in your zone, your imagination having rehearsed and now perfuming, your thoughts flow one after the other, as you feel so very peaceful, almost like you have been at this for sixteen to nineteen years. Your mind so clever and adaptive, your mind and your speech, so free flowing, nuances start to bubble up to the surface, all that you share and express so very cohesive.

Your correct response to any and all stress is to deep breathe, relax, and see any opportunity of expressing yourself as a time to play, a time to perform, for all that the seasoned professionals do and know, so now you know and do.

You speak from your ribs and your stomach, you modulate well, joyously express, and your audience expresses appreciation regarding what you have to say.

You find joy in what you are doing and how you are expressing yourself.

You share the excitement and enjoy, and it's just getting easier and more successful, you succeeding easily, while relaxing into a perfumer's flow, your enthusiasm is infectious.

What anyone thinks of you is none of your business, you are there to share, to teach, mightier and greater than any and all challenges, for the greater the challenge, the greater and mightier you are, and simply in all moments of presenting, your inner entertainer rising to the top, successfully switched on, you now learning or succeeding, so at home in front of an audience, so ready to present, play and have fun.

Becoming a Master Public Speaker

Each and every time you're in front of an audience to speak, whether it's to one or two people or a large crowd, even in front of any media, you are so supported and comfortable, so at ease, completely relaxed, your inner performer rises to the top, activated, thriving from the experience of your powerfully effective many years of doing this.

All of your very best abilities come together, as the words flow from you, like an unstoppable river of energy, from heart and mind, with ease, free of effort, getting any and all of your points across smoothly, with maximum clarity, brightly, as your mighty inner hero, and greatest communicator, speaks articulately, in a free flow, with confidence and clarity, anxiety free, comfortable, as if playing a role.

As if your talented mighty inner entertainer has risen to the top, playful, reassured, self encouraged, feeling the audiences support of you, their thirst for knowledge, their desire for the information you impart, you as their teacher, sharing information, and enlightenment, you now, in a brand new chapter of your life, all things reset, re-tuned, retained, recalibrated, all things unpleasant or uncomfortable now released into now and forever done past chapters of your life.

You now fortified and adaptive, relaxed and thriving, embraced, supported and inspired by the energy of every past victory, triumph, breakthrough and success you've ever had or even imagined having.

Blockage free, free flowing, moving onward, unbeatable, free of second guessing, flowing and thriving, clear and on the path, flowing yet structured, able to change pace, make a joke, change and enhance the energy, precise, free of struggling or trying, simply getting the job done.

Your mind free flowing, clear and laser-beam precise, so very sharp, your memory fine-tuned, as you more easily than ever before draw upon your knowledge and experience of the last [7, 10, 22, 35] years, while easily able to remember, perform, recall, and even present it all to others effectively and concisely, by understanding the lay of the land and landscape, almost as if you have done the equivalent of eight to sixteen years worth of improving yourself in this area, as you are and you remain, doing even better each and every time you repeat this wonderful technique upon your own.

Slipping into deepest levels of relaxation, inspiration, activation, and realization, while your comfortable body and all of its melted and relaxed muscles, as well as your emotions, your thoughts, so serene, so peaceful, so ready, so relaxed, so easily stepping up to meet any and all challenges, most especially whenever challenged to perform, you just doing better and better, in ways both known and unknown to you.

In fact or just truly, it all seems to be, foundationally restructured, as you are now and forever putting this together, better than ever before.

Any and all of this, not because I say so, but because it is in fact true, you sense it, you feel it, and you now truly and forever know it, as you are now living within it, any and all of this now, enhanced, easier and better, all around you.

In your mind, you now know, from foundational places deepest inside of you, that you are and you remain a more interested and focused, a better public and even private speaker, a voracious success with large and small groups, at anything and every thing you put your mind to.

Self-Confidence and Public Speaking – Corporate

In this moment of deep and truly profound relaxation, you have relaxed your way into a brand new and better chapter in your life.

Perhaps it's only your imagination, or maybe it's even true, for you have done fifteen to eighteen years worth of healing, in this moment, as well as in each and every moment that you repeat this wonderfully enjoyable technique on your own.

In this place of deep and profound relaxation, you are activating from deep, deep within yourself the ability to generate limitless strength and confidence while speaking with anyone or in front of groups in public, easily speaking your mind allowing inner wisdom to generate and flow from each and every word, each and every movement of your body, each and every posture and movement, each and every gesture with your body or your hands.

In this brand new and better chapter of your life, the harmony of heart and mind generating in your wisdom, now bubbles up the surface, whenever you need it, as your breathing is deep, and serene, and peaceful, as you remain comfortable and stress-free, and everything just seems to flow, free of over-thinking, you are simply in the moment allowing all of this to happen.

Not because I say so, but because in fact you have reset something from deep inside of you, perhaps a switch, a dial, thermostat of some kind, or even a computer that generates limitless and endless success.

Your correct response to any and all stress is to relax your way through it by deep breathing, and relaxing your way beyond, trusting in your life and what you have to say or present to others.

For you now believe in yourself, but beyond belief there is faith, and beyond faith there is knowing, and you simply now know that you are coming together in this process of unlimited healing in the most high-impact and profound ways possible, doing better and better, relaxing in to a better flow of life.

You are very relaxed at work, always remaining stress-free, even when speaking with others in important situations.

You are problem-free and challenge-oriented from now on, all of this getting better and easier for you - for the more challenging the situation, the more you rise up to meet it, greet it and effectively and inspirationally deal with it, to ultimate success.

Now and in the future, you have accepted, embraced, and risen up mightily to enhance this new and always working in your favor to limitless success profound truth.

You face any and all challenging situations by running at them directly, more easily confident in your knowledge and abilities than ever before.

In this brand new and better chapter of your life, you are free of using cigarettes or food as a crutch.

You are doing so much better by deciding to always treat yourself in the ways you know you must, to take the very best care of yourself, easily rising up skillfully, and with the skill of a master at any and all of this, for what they know, you know, for what they do, you do, for what they have become, you now and forever are.

Certain and sure of this, you are unstoppable and unbeatable, and all that you focus your mind upon, easily rising up in any moment you need to, for in fact truly, this is what you will always do.

At night while you rest, you allow your day to be put up on the shelf, resting peacefully at night, sleeping peacefully right through the night, falling back to sleep as quickly as you need to, pleasant happy dreams inspire and support you.

Your life now reorganized, you now so motivated, mighty, capable, happy and even heroic.

You're taking the very best care of yourself with exercise, and your appearance, leading a more organized life, treating yourself better and better as a natural extension of all of this, in ways both known and unknown to you, motivationally and unstoppably driven to succeed in your life.

Not because I say so but is because it is the nature of your own mind, body, the motions, an inner wisdom to do so, and therefore it is and remains forever, almost as if the large burden has been lifted off you once and forever, and for always, you have unbeatably succeeded here, and feel pride in heart mind having done so.

Any and all of this becoming easier and better, more adaptive, and skillfully created for you. Deep breath detaching you from stressful moments, creating a centered feeling from deep within.

Slowly consumed better meals taking better care of you, you taking the very best care of yourself, even feeling so inspired to breakthrough here.

All of this triggering pleasant and happy embracing feelings and memories almost as if being as carefree as when you were in 6th grade summer camp, knowing that for all of summer worry free experiencing only happiness.

Living A Better Dream: Success, Self-Confidence and Procrastination Free

You have relaxed and floated and drifted and dreamed your way into a brand new chapter of your life.

You are now determined, more than ever before to create a masterpiece of life, the kind you always envisioned, the kind you know you deserve, the kind that you dynamically and easily create to be true to yourself, and all of those you love and care about.

For beyond belief, there is faith, and beyond faith, there is simply knowing, knowing who you are, respecting yourself, and realizing that you are the best in the world you have to offer anyone, so all of you now is foundationally reset, re-tuned, recalibrated, thrivingly so and alive, feeling inspired while generating confidence, and knowing who you are.

Any and all of this is becoming better and easier, by setting up your place to effectively and easily, in your life, get the job done.

You schedule out what it is you need to do, you respect yourself by going to bed early enough, sleeping deeply, peacefully, while receiving inspirational dreams, to get the job done, both skillfully and effectively.

In all you do, you have relaxed beyond all former and now done barriers in your life, to handle your life better, most assuredly better, to take better care of your finances and yourself better, respecting yourself, as if having grown up just a little bit more, which is all it really takes and all it will really take in any moment, most especially whenever challenged.

It has been said, there is no trying, there is either not doing or doing, so you most effectively and cleverly do, and create and inspirationally generate, as you now know you succeed, you break through, you are more motivated, finding reasons and inspirations, more focused than ever before to get this done, while liberating a future moment of success, that is gloriously yours right now, into the right here and now.

Your days of trying and struggling are now at an end, each and every little step forward, leads to a greater and more significant breakthrough, even if the times that seems not to make any sense, any and all of this, is now generating, more precise and measured success in each and every moment.

Your imagination allows you to dream up new plans, while circumventing roadblocks from now done chapters in the past, generating inner as well as outer fulfillment and achieving your dreams, making anything and everything you desire to achieve your own.

Not because I say so, but because it is the nature of your own mind to do this. And so it is, and so it gets done.

For anything to happen in life, there's a *thought* or an *idea.* These now more easily formulate in your mind into your actions and your thoughts, and your feelings, as a *plan,* as every heartbeat and breath now moves you forward into activating a now noticeably better and more effectively functional reality around yourself, generating correct and precise action to accomplish any and all desired goals, while skillfully avoiding pitfalls, rising to the top, activating inner wisdom and divine guidance, to get the job done.

Any task at hand, you now an unstoppable force, and all you seek to achieve, and so it is, and actively remains, on each and every breath, and on each and every heartbeat, with every blink of your eyes, each and every day, each and every night, all of you, body, emotions, mind, even spirit, achieve a more dynamic harmony and life-force, pushing you forward into your life.

Even while you dream at night, fulfilling, happy dreams, allowing you to work out issues, feeling so very inspired in the morning, and more super motivated, to seize the day, get any and all jobs done.

You know, it's almost as if someone from deep, deep inside of you has reset the switch, the dial, a thermostat, or activated the computer of some kind, so that everything works together in your favor.

All of this seems to be happening around you, as you have set this into motion, feeling this and knowing this as a new and improved truth, knowing it as real, and having given this life, which generates results both complete, motivated, and exciting to you, in the most profoundly effective of ways, all of this worked out.

You generate support and inspiration for yourself far more easily and more freely until it becomes a habit.

Now and forever knowing, you are clever, clear, sharp, and more highly skilled and effective at this, the more you know it, and the more you do it, a happier as the more motivated you become.

You now enrich yourself mentally and emotionally, even spiritually, as you are and as you remain providing this for yourself, even reinventing yourself as you need to, to do all that it takes to actualize and to break through, thrive, and succeed.

Taking even better care of yourself becomes easier and better for you, as new mightier habits and reactions now emerge, and you are now more certain, peaceful, serene, and sure of yourself than ever before in your life.

You are now foundationally readjusted into a better moment of your life, instilled with a sense of inner peace and truth, that makes any and all of this more unstoppably so.

Energized, Moving Forward

You are now and you remain more fearless and dynamic than ever before.

Your mighty inner hero now rises to the top here and forever, almost as if having thrown a switch, a dial, a thermostat, or computer into action, that will forever effectively work out as well as completely alleviate, any and all details of breaking through here and free you unbeatably.

You begin to relax, enjoy the experience of exercise, almost like having begun a brand new chapter of your life, where you are free, clear and healed.

Any and all things that ever once stood in your way, a now removed and pushed out, now in a done and finished chapter of your life.

Just relax and succeed. As you relax deeper and further, you become your true self, more dynamic, mighty, more who you used to be, except now, even better, sharper, smarter, and more unbeatable, in anything and everything you set your mind to.

Your breath and your legs work to carry you into this brand new chapter of your life, free at long last, it feels great to be so free, almost like you're bathing in a healing energetic sea of relaxation and freedom.

Each and every little step forward means a lot, as you step into each and every moment of your life with every movement of your legs, and your body, every thought and desire that you wish to achieve now becomes more your own, as you completely in forever transcend the past, you are now truly free on each and every breath, every slow and steady heartbeat, your body and mind, even your emotions, now rebalanced, retained, reset, in ways most effective and unlimited.

Self-Confidence in Social Situations

You always knew that someday your life would improve, and right now is that moment of power.

You relax, see, imagine, or just simply truly know, now is the time to rise to the top and relax beyond former barriers and become mighty.

And so you are and now do, as you relax even deeper and further, letting it all go, deeper and further it's almost as if someone from deep inside of you has accelerated your growth and healing process [twelve to seventeen] years, having reset a switch, a dial, a thermostat of some kind.

Easily allowing you to find it very free-flowing and more easily able to approach people, especially [beautiful women, handsome men] and strike up a conversation, because you are more and more sharing something of the most valuable asset you have in your life, you!

So much more and more appealing, outgoing and inspired, brimming with knowing and glowing confidence, winning confidence, a source of incredible power for you, now yours forever.

Almost like you have matured many years, you are and you remain solid yet flexible knowing who you are, taking life and more of a flow, so knowing who you are, inspired by your mighty inner hero, you are free of letting anything get to you, for the more challenging the situation, the better you feel inside, stronger and more focused.

In situations once found challenging by you, you relax, speak your heart and mind, all of this becomes second nature to you, calm and cool, your strong and steady heart rate, comfortable, life supporting breathing, rhythm, flowing, skin temperature, all working non stop in your favor, as your automatic mind now works up methods, strategies, social skills, and solutions to break a through, in ways both known and even unknown to you.

You also learn to start conversations and become a wonderful listener, most especially when it comes [women, men].

You truly come to know, your whole presence now like a giant magnet of some kind, easily engaging, illuminating and attracting business prospects, friends, and most especially [women, men].

You relax deeper, you foundationally know this to be true.

Where in the past you may have frozen up, right now your automatic dynamic mind is working out ways for you to become more comfortable in any situation or place as you become and remain more and more sociable and able to free flowingly communicate.

You adapt, and with a winning attitude, almost like the world is yours, all things working out in balance, you now at a better more supportive pace, you seize the moment.

What others think of you is none of your business.

Your correct and proper response to challenge, is a calm and relaxed attitude. You learn to love yourself first, and present a strong relaxed comfortable presence and demeanor to all people and situations you may encounter.

Being shy was yesterday, and you now know that yesterday is over.

Now a true, sure and certain, completely positive, serene and confident, mature, a new day has dawned in your life, a happier and better night for you.

You now relax, you give up trying, you simply are, be and do. In this moment, so relaxed, a blanket of energy around you, you trust in life.

You relax and become one with the world around you, free of struggling or trying, those moments now done and gone forever, whether you yet realize it at this moment or at some point in the future, or just now as it now dawns upon you, feeling and knowing it,. you become more at one with all people in the world, you were meant to be here, a valuable friend and asset to everyone you know.

You learn to love yourself better and more, restored and mighty, now unstoppable.

Positively and absolutely determined to release self condemnation, better instead self-supporting, the past is now done, you love and respect yourself so much more, boldly stepping into today and tomorrow, yesterday now done forever, feeling great to be so freed.

Free from the damage inflicted by others, your opinion of yourself the only important thing. Loving yourself enough to release, heal, and forgive the past, you're doing so much better, what other people think of you is none of your business.

You begin to treat yourself like some somebody you love and care about.

You relax and decide to polish yourself and become brilliant, relax, at times as needed, free-flowing, aloof, mysterious, confident, free flowing speech, all the things you seek are inside of you, all of you enough, all of you knitting back together again, or just even better, almost like you have surely done the equivalent of twelve to seventeen years of life improvement, all of this getting even better and more pronounced, more high-Impact, adaptive, and flexible, each and every time you reinforce this on your own.

You run your own race, you take your own pace, you find your own place; you simply know you are just doing better and better.

Want and need and is now forgiven and released, relaxed away from and moved into the past, beyond belief. You simply know who you are, you are enough, the center of your own world, relaxed in your own skin, as it is all coming together on your own.

Able to set boundaries more easily, standing up for yourself, taking the very best care of yourself.

You learn being kind yourself and taking things in stride, work out so much better for you until it ends in perfection, perfection is contained within, you write your perfection on the surface, so whether flawed or perfected, you are enough, loving yourself enough to know this to be the truth.

You resolve right here and now, to treat yourself better, and as you do, on every breath and heartbeat, you notice it, as the world begins to know this new you emerging, you're respected, and more comfortable in your own skin, all issues working themselves out and ways very best, both known and unknown to you.

The very best opinion of yourself is yours. The most important person you have to respect is you, so true, you do.

The most important opinions about life are yours. Loving yourself enough to give yourself a break, you break through unbeatably.

Liking and loving yourself enough, you become an endless reservoir of self respect, confident and clear, as well as loved, and self-loved while, forever free of struggling or trying, you simply are, and loved, as the world takes notice, and is attracted to you magnetically.

Sales/Healthy Living/Life Motivation

You have forever entered brand new chapter of your life.

All of the adjustments necessary, all of the tweaks, any and all things necessary, have been reset, re-tuned, redefined, and improved in your favor.

You know this to be true because it is, from the deepest recesses inside of you.

Each and every aspect and area of your life, now working in a greater higher harmony, as the heroic and mighty inner master of your life, that you are, from deepest places inside, is now automatically allowing this to happen, skillfully adjusting and adapting, only your very best, ways that serve you best and for those that you love the most, most especially yourself.

In this newer and brighter, better chapter of your life, you are re-excited about things, easily adapting to each and every challenge, for the mightier than challenge, the more clever, adaptive, and intense, you are in the most propitious of ways.

On the phone, your excitement about anything and everything you have to share, easily spreads, infectiously, and the very best of ways, to other people, knowing what you share is of great value, and importance, relaxed, the getting all points across clearly.

Hearing, "I don't know" or "I don't care" on the other end of the phone, means please explain it better to me, and make me understand.

Every no, is only one step closer to a yes, every no, even moment of hesitation or apathy, on the part of the other person, means please make me understand.

You begin to think in new and better ways, for you believe in yourself.

But beyond belief, there is faith, and beyond faith there is knowingness, as your automatic mind begins to work out a better day, a better night, a more graceful approach to your life, better and more balanced life supporting impulses, easily work out for you to unbeatably regain intensity, as you are now redefined.

You begin to enjoy a greater ease within your life, and a greater joy of movement, once set in motion, the more easily you are able to move forward, sticking with the exercise plan, making this time just for you.

As a way of loving yourself more, loving yourself better, you begin to work out, and find reasons and even excuses to get that done.

Your tastes and impulses improved in your favor.

You begin to eat better every day as you exercise more, taking better care of yourself, you fill up sooner, a small taste is enough for you, you savor the taste, smells, and sensations, just a small taste of sugar, dairy, carbohydrates, are enough to you.

You begin to front load your carbohydrates earlier in the day, allowing brain function, eating a higher protein base later in the day, taking even better care of yourself.

You maintain vitamin levels, electrolytes, and drink plenty of water, washing you clean inside, making better choices, less is more, you fill up sooner, you doing better, sleeping peacefully right through the night, any and all of this allowing a better night's rest, peaceful and happy dreams, and those dreams work out any and all issues, as your life seems to be improving, automatically.

Life Motivation - 1

In these profound moments of deeper and ever more soothing relaxation, in these moments of profound and healing rejuvenation, somehow you just now know you are and you remain relaxing deeper and further on each and every breath you take, and on each and every heartbeat, and as you do, you flow, event, and drift, flowing ever onward and beyond, any and all now released and former vanquished obstacles or blockages, so now and forever done, into a brand new chapter of your life.

Harmonized, healing, whole, healed, reset, reaching ever higher and higher, only to your very best, re-tuned, recalibrated, almost as if each and every issue you once found challenging, almost as if each challenge, is now removed, having been learned from, and therefore released, and risen above,.

You now and forever, so much more now knitted back together again, and moving beyond.

Polished, seasoned, shinier, better than ever, better than new, as you do, as you are, it is almost as if you have relaxed right now, as you will relax like this in the future, even deeper and greater in fact.

All things once in disharmony are now actively and adaptively forever now reset, and re-tuned, recalibrated, all of you completely improved, for beyond belief is faith, and beyond that, there is simply knowing, now knowing, your greatest place of inspirational power and success.

And as you now completely and truly forever now know, who you are, and as you are growing, you are improving, yet however, now more than ever, knowing who you are, truly, you now enough are, as yourself esteem and self confidence now radiates, from this knowledge, seemingly, all of your life, released and improving, unbeatably in your favor.

Each and every anything that you set your mind to, you become more passionate about, each and every passion, you now focus upon by the conquering, or just simply get powerfully making any and all of this your own as you are now and forever cleverly and adaptively, becoming one with, including, anxiety release, better time management, reinstatement and reactivation of both memory and recall, all of that by simply relaxing, some very truly and deeply inspired, all of your ambitions, now so much more easily your very own.

Your self esteem & self confidence rise, re-tune and reset, feeling this profoundly in heart and mind, as a glowing happy warmth.

The past is now the past, on each and every breath, and each and every heartbeat, waves of forgiveness and release now become apparent as you feel or even just simply imagine, the release and letting go, not only of harsh judgments of others, but even more so than more specialty, for yourself, off yourself, forgiving and releasing, even healing, in the most profound of ways.

It's almost as if a light from above shines down upon you from somewhere, generating limitless healing, release, and forgiveness, not because I say so, but because it is in the nature of things, that it is so, accelerating your healing process, the equivalent of four, nine, fifteen to eighteen years, each and every time you do this with even greater impact in benefit on your own.

All that you wish to be, all that you aspire to become, you now step forward into, forever into a brand new chapter of your life, rejuvenated, reset, and reconditioned, all that you are excited by, you honestly step forward and generate all appropriate energy, magnetizing opportunities, while activating action, reaction, motivation and inspiration, all everything and anything to most effectively get the job done.

Liberating only your very best, your very best days and nights, you now generate, finding even interest and fascination and things you once found challenging, loving every moment of your life, almighty are the challenge for more motivated you become while enjoying support, more unconditional love, and greater moments of happiness, so very well deserved, so very much more now your own.

Life Motivation - 2

As you relax, float, drift, and dream, you relax, flow and float beyond any and all now done and former limits into a better chapter of your life.

You relax deeper, as the procrastination melts away, as you are now so unstoppably determined to [go back to school, get a better job, save money, etc].

Your mind relaxes, you calm down, your mind opens, you remember some time in your life feelings super inspired, that inspiration is yours now, as you're now opened and ready to assimilate mind, greatly accelerates your learning ability and enjoyment for learning, and only the very best of ways, highly effective and precise ways, in ways both known and unknown to you.

Achieving this you do, as much as possible.

New ideas, thoughts, inspirations, and methods of success now become one with you, your mind relaxes, a new chapter begins, all of it coming together on its own.

Doing any and all of this, each and every method and technique, more and more extremely useful, in powerful yet beneficial ways.

In this new chapter of your life, you are forgiven, healed and released, finding a new thriving, an abiding sense of inner peace, calmness and inner quiet, becoming more and more whole-minded, mentally quiet and focused, very gently and dynamically, coming to a place of peace and release, that easily forever vanquishes any internal conflict, you now more single minded and focused, easily achieving beneficial results.

All of this now allowing you to achieve better dreams, inspirations, motivations, and successes, even feeling a shift of energy all around you right now, more certain and sure of this you are now than ever before in your life.

Living in energized focus, more relaxed, you easily achieved your dreams, and while resting at night, almost as if an aspect of you has been kicked into some higher gear, you lucidly dream more easily.

Your body relaxes, your mind's eye clear and sharp, thoughts clear and focused, yet relaxed, achieving hassle-free focus better, and with greater results, getting into the emptiness easily and longer, the empty vessel you are, able to be fulfilled finally.

In fact, truly, a new you rises up mightily, and ready to thrive, you begin, almost anew, reset, restarted, recalibrated, socially magnetic, passionate and dynamic, letting your inner hero awaken and rise up, so inspired, doing only better and better for yourself and those you love most, more and most especially for yourself.

Intrepid, courageous, bold, dynamic, mighty, magnetizing only the very best, repelling all the rest, truly now knowing this feeling of yourself driven and empowered, inspired, like a force of nature, unstoppable, focused, spirited, audacious.

Now knowing any and all of this to be true, rising up to meet your higher purpose, and life's purpose, new inspirations and talents arise, driving you forward, trusting in the fact that your life is working out in your favor and you are making it happen.

Your very best thoughts activate, as you see something of yourself in all things and all people, circumstances, and events, you so inspired, all proper thoughts and inspirations at just the rightist moments, on their own, bringing in the harvest of manifestation, to the benefit of all those you know and yourself.

For in past chapters of your life, the blockages once there, are and now and forever turned around to break you through here, and are now used as fuel, even firewood.

Their now empowering energy, now used to propel you forward into the kind of a life and world, filled with more joy, life, enjoyment, security, brilliance, energy, focus and motivation, to propel you forward into the kind of a masterpiece life you now generate and enjoy the benefits from.

You magnetize all you need to support yourself in more balanced, effective and brilliant ways, and repel the rest, generating only all of the very best!

Life Improvement
– Concentration, Anger Release, Better Life

In this brand new and better chapter of your life you are more easily and exceptionally breaking though into your very, very best, having grown up just a bit more.

Disinterest and disgust are now lifting, going, going and gone, far, far away from you, as you always knew,this would get done and be easier and better as your life went on, and so it is and begins now, almost as if someone from deep, deep, inside of you, has reset a switch, a dial a thermostat or a computer of some kind, easily and yet powerfully, resetting, feeling that energy leave, and as focus now more and more becomes a permanent and real part of you.

You are doing better, more and more willing to rise up and become the person you were best meant to be and are now more and more willing to take charge and become, not because I say so, but because it is in fact the nature of whom you are really are and were meant to be.

You now listen to your own inner voice and reason what needs to be, the limitations and limiting opinions of others, so much now less important to you.

As you relax deeper and further, your mind now so relaxed, now so clear, so much more serene and peaceful, fortified, easily able to, in ways both known and unknown to you, rise above any and all obstacles and breakthrough here, even simply just able to focus and concentrate.

Breaking through here better and truer to yourself, a more successful chapter of your life, more easily able and enabled to focus and concentrate, and recall, remember and perform with ease, skill and strength, for the more you know and love all of whom you are, the more and more easily able you are to focus and concentrate.

Finding inner harmony, a wisdom begins to light up, burn and remove any and all darkness, as you now, right now, more calm and more serene, almost as if these calming and soothing relaxation feelings are staying with you from these moments and are now becoming a permanent and real, true part of you.

For the calmer and more peaceful you are and become, the greater your life and happiness.

You are in fact in a brand new and better chapter of your life and your existence, having grown up just a bit more, now knowing that the best ways to control is to relax, let go, flow, and now feeling from memory a time of profound rest and peace, you now more easily choose to be better and more calm, more self-appreciative and self-loving, knowing that your very best is rising to the very top and are now more and more easily finding newer and better ways of breaking yourself through, to be a happier and better you.

Creating for yourself a breakthrough, so much better and more peaceful, happier, just right for you.

You are simply done with trying to get it right and are just getting it right, right now, self-forgiven, releasing, released, letting out your better and your very best.

Done with all unpleasantness, hatred, hostility, anger. All are powerfully forgotten and forgiven, and forgiving, releasing, released, releasing and more and more whole, forgetting, and simply in a brand new and reconditioned, better chapter of your life.

Truly, all of your existence, finding and creating ways to love, and understand, be loved, and understood, and become one with your life and those you love most, most especially yourself, more with yourself and others, more one on one and appreciating yourself and others, creating a masterpiece of a life and lifetime more now than ever before.

Your past now shed, a new and more successful chapter of your life and your world now more and more easily yours and your own.

All things that once stood in your way, now out of your way, out of your way, you now are and more easily enabled to set aside things once held onto, to become more and more free as you need to be, to succeed here and forever, your mighty and unstoppable dynamic mind, now more and more easily generating this automatically, sharing all of only your very best, releasing and forgiving.

Your mind now calm and clear, focused, information and thought, now coming and going, trusting your first and better instincts, your concentration now laser beam like precise in anything and everything you need to accomplish, for the mightier the task, the more and more inspired, powerful and able, enabled you are and you become.

You either breakthrough here, or simply, just succeed!

Better English Speaking Hypnotist, Fear Free, Money Magnet

As you relax deeper and further, further and deeper, your mind relaxes and yet rises up to be heroic and mighty, to clear and release any and all things from now finished past and done chapters of your life.

Just visualize, picture, sense, imagine, or perhaps really, truly even know, that it's almost like you've done the equivalent of twelve to seventeen years worth of work and experience in practicing English in this moment, and in each and every moment which you choose to practice Self-Hypnosis in this way.

As your mind now relaxes and clears, you are completely open and absolutely ready to learn, take on new things, coalesce yourself into being a better hypnotist than even you have ever imagined, become a master of suggestion writing.

In fact, in each and every way, you are doing better and better, for all things that you were once afraid of now seem to be melting away, and draining away far, far away from you, almost like growing up into adulthood, free of childish ways, owning your responsibilities and life.

For within you, a sense of everyone else, in everyone else, a part of you.

You trust inwardly and outside of you, all things are working unstoppably in your favor, to allow you to become in forever remain, 100% fluent listening, speaking and understanding.

Your life, your creation, your life, a place you create and trust.

It is almost like within your mind, someone has reset the switch, a dial, a valve, or computer of some kind, that allows you to rise up and become mighty, barrier free, free of past self-criticism, trusting in your life, frustrations-free, powerful and trusting, fearless and mighty, driven and focused on enough to be only at your very best, failure free, choosing to learn or succeed unbeatably.

Re-tuned, reset, rejuvenated, you re-identify yourself as a powerful hypnotist, easily becoming one of the very best there is in your homeland, or anywhere you go.

For in this new and better chapter of your life, you choose to either learn or succeed, and so you do.

Being driven, focused, unbeatable, your mind works unstoppably in your favor while you are awake, while you are asleep, even while you dream, to set all of this up so well deserved and happily.

Any and all parts of your life, now resetting and returning themselves to break you through here.

Your mind now expands about finances and money, you know sense, picture, or even see money as a source of energy, as you put out joy and productive work into the world, as a form of energy, so too does the energy of money, coming back to you.

For beyond belief there is faith, beyond faith, now you simply know, your relationship with finances and money are now retuning anything and everything, to allow your heart and mind to light up and restore you as a money magnet.

The Divine aspect within you, is now open to the resource of abundance, dynamically, for the Divine within you, deserves it.

As you now know a new chapter of your life has begun, you know take better care of yourself, feeling free and safe, deeply and truly now and forever know you can accomplish anything and everything you need, deserve, or want.

Reaching every one of your goals easily and with great dynamic impact and success.

Anytime you and I work together, and I ask you to relax and say strongly the word *sleep*, your whole body becomes loose, limp, and relaxed, your mind relaxes, your body relaxes, and you instantly drop into a deep and restful relaxation trance state, wide open to any and all improvements and suggestions only in the very best of ways, You and I working together as a team.

Your powerful subconscious mind is your friend working in your favor, for all things once working against you are released and reversed, goals now more and more easily set and achieved, you and your mind, working in a harmony and in concert, you now you, your very own best friend.

Better Self-Esteem and Goal Setting

You relax and now come to know that you have completely and successfully entered a new chapter of your life, and come to an understanding that you have moved into a better constructed and more self-supporting, believing in yourself and moreover, knowing who you are and loving yourself enough, to elevate yourself.

Give yourself a break, become mightier and mightier within yourself to surmount the past and rise up, becoming mightier than any challenge in your memory or in your life, as you believe in yourself.

But beyond belief, there is faith, hope and the charity you bring to yourself a newer and greater belief, in all that you are and in all that you do.

Beyond thinking, there is a newer way, and now you are simply knowing, who you are, and you, this powerful you, is doing better and better at your life.

You begin to think in new and better, more and more self-supporting ways, taking things in stride, relaxing beyond now done, outdated, outgrown and done, former barriers, released and forgiven into past chapters of your life only.

Making a better day, a better way, a better night, patiently, and at a better pace, setting up schedules and plans that suit you, fluidly and adaptively yet, sticking to a schedule to get the job done clearly, actively, and efficiently.

You develop and learn to set goals and to please yourself with the results, always allowing more room for improvement, for the more pleased you are with yourself, the more people around you are also pleased.

You do everything and anything that it takes to honestly and effectively get the job done, while taking things in stride, even relaxing and flowing beyond barriers, your thought pattern shifting into a pattern more suitable for you and in the very best of ways.

You strive only for the very best, you are happy with realistic results.

The more at home within yourself, the more comfortable within your skin.

So you relax, memorizing the feelings and sensations, so easily recreated, almost like you've grown up another sixteen to eighteen years, trusting in your life, and doing all that it takes to effectively and completely live your life as an adult.

Doing all it takes to honestly succeed and breakthrough, standing tall, even allowing yourself to feel proud about the things you've done and accomplished, as you love yourself more, you know who you are, and live a better life.

You begin to forgive and release any repetition about the past moments of your life that ever once stood in your way, in ways both known and unknown to you, for every time you nod your head Yes you are saying yes to the very best that life can bring you.

Ahhhh, it feels so great to be so free.

You come to a greater place of wisdom and self truth in your life.

You remain adaptive yet unshakable in this, each and every day, no matter what the challenge.

While there is always room for improvement, you do it in a self-loving way, reinventing how you communicate to yourself internally taking things in a better normal stride, realizing you are important and you were meant to be here.

For the more challenging the situation is, the more challenging the person is, has been, or will be, from your past, present, or future, you are more calm, centered, peaceful, relaxed, out of your own way, rising above, and whether you were aware of it or not, feeling more support from yourself and the universe around you in general, to allow you to get the jobs done in your life.

Trusting in your life, you are sleeping peacefully each and every night, waking up in the morning more comfortable in your life, more comfortable in your skin, generally knowing that you are doing anything and everything it honestly takes in ways known and unknown to you, to forgive, to heal, to coalesce, refine, polish and improve anything and everything within you, to love yourself enough to break through into the very best, shiniest, brightest, better, most successful chapter of your life, even beyond your wildest dreams and anticipations.

You take things in a more calm and more wonderful stride, getting the job done.

Any and all of this working in your favor, not because I say so, but because it is within the nature of your own mind, emotions, thoughts, inspirations, feelings, even spirit, and wise inner hero, to get this done.

All things are working out better and better for you, whether it's scheduling, goal completion, each and every little step forward meaning a lot as you get to the finish line.

Believing in and knowing who you are as a capable and loving person, trusting in your life that all things, big or small, known or as yet unknown, are working out in their own way to your maximum benefit, for the greater the challenge, the mightier and more inspired and empowered you become.

Each and every thought, each and every feeling, realigning, generates known feelings and expressions of freedom within you, and your heart now glows in a warm light, the energy reaches and connects to your thoughts generating a greater sense of peacefulness and wisdom within you.

Life Support

You decide to rise up and become mighty, you rise up, now more powerful and capable, ready to handle anything, taking slower, slower and steady and more relaxing deep breaths, all things once limiting to you, now a thing of the past, you now the mighty heroic one in your life, and giving yourself credit for being who you really are, more unlimited, more unstoppable, more fluid and dynamic, more unbeatable, more easily able, to rise above any limitation or challenge, for the mightier than challenge, the more inspired, dynamic, empowered, enabled, resourceful, and powerful you become, as you now take deep and steady breath, now releasing any and all imbalance, rhythmically and ideally, leaving a noticeable and yet unstoppable feeling of serenity deep inside of you.

Much like being alongside the still waters of a serene and calming mountain lake, your adaptive, fluid, and unstoppable creative mind, now creates, habits, ideas, strategies, solutions, to remove clutter, calm chatter, and you know beyond all things, you are fully enabled to do each and every thing, anything and everything, it takes for you to breakthrough, thrive and succeed.

Not because I say so, but it is in fact because the nature of your own mind, and your unstoppable, divinely guided, indelible spirit, will create, only balance and harmony, heroically, in this brand new and better chapter of your life.

You now know this to be true, not because I say so, but because, you have been reset, re-tuned, recalibrated, and are truly unbeatable and any and all of this, relaxed, trusting in your abilities and your life, now knowing you will be better than okay, even just fine.

You are truly in fact, in this brand new chapter of your life, beginning to better create a life, and a map, and a plan, with every habit, action, reaction, so very fluidly adaptive, to now trust in yourself and your life, and in the way it is unfolding.

You now rising to the occasion, better now than ever before, knowing that you are bigger and mightier than any challenge ever presented to you in your life, you now overwhelming the challenges, as you now are and recognize yourself as always having been.

Recognizing and appreciating yourself for who you truly are and will always be, heroic and mighty, adaptive, successful, fluid and creative, as you rise up, as a truly unstoppable force of light and healing.

For the greater the challenge, the more determined, even stubborn and obstinate to achieve success as you now let yourself loose to fully become to see it, any and all of it, through to the very end.

When the day is over, an hour or so before bedtime, you choose to put the day upon a shelf, relax all over, unwind, deep breathe, slow and steady breath, soothing you and

180

healing you, in both body, mind, emotions, and in fact all that you very are, feeling more steady and more stable, so that when it is time for bed, tonight and each and every other night, and from now on always in this new chapter of your life, you have only put your head on the pillow, close your eyes, and go to sleep.

It is simply that easy, to sleep so much better through the night, resting comfortably through the night, almost as if someone from deep, deep inside of you, has reset a switch, a dial, or thermostat of some kind, having re-tuned you, reset you, restored you, recalibrated you, very best of ways, in ways most relaxing, fluid yet fortified, your mind more relaxed, thoughts becoming like vapor drifting away from you.

Your emotions and your mind so much more now very calm, new habits and skills for relaxation, rest and success now and forever yours, in ways both known and unknown, where you will either, thrive or succeeded unbeatably, or simply become part of the new chapter of your life.

So at each and every bedtime, you right there, more drowsy, more weary, unwinding, heavy, thought and relaxation drifting, more trusting in your life, than ever before in your life, most especially when you are ready to fall asleep at night, each and every night, more peacefully and easily sleeping through the night, even more fully rested when it's time to wake up in the morning, even if it's a short night of sleep, just a few hours, more fully refreshing, more rejuvenating, more inspiring an empowering to you, then ever before.

It has been said that belief is a very powerful thing.

Beyond belief, there is faith, even more powerful, beyond faith, there is simply knowing, the most powerful of all, and in this new and more improved, self-supporting, self-loving chapter of your life, more self-forgiving and self-loving, you now know who you are, powerful, a good person, there are for others, more so now, better, therefore you, loving yourself, filling yourself up, goodness from deep, deep within.

Trusting in your life and yourself, to be in abundant supply, for everyone and anybody, that may need your assistance, until the day is done, handling any and all circumstances, with the skill of a master, as you have always done, except this time, knowing that important fact, and arriving unlimited strength and resourcefulness, from that fact.

Whether at home or at work, whether working for yourself or others, in fact in any and all relationships, you're simply doing better and better for yourself, and for all concerned, because you can actually feel, you actually now notice, you actually now remember, that can-do spirit and energy, of the dynamic and mighty hero that resides within you.
In the very best of ways, both fluid and adaptive, and the very best of ways both known and unknown to you, in this brand new chapter of your life, much like letting go of the habits and reactions of the child you once were, so to now and forever in this moment do you improve dramatically.

In this brand new and better, chapter of your life, improvements happen more rapidly as barriers from the past now seem to be falling away, evaporating, vanquished, the light of your heart and mind, working in harmony to vanquish forever the shadows, releasing imbalances, forgiving and letting go of old and useless no longer wanted habits you are now and forever free from, finding calmness, truly tranquility and inner peace.

You find joy in more simple things, taking little breaks mean a lot, find yourself laughing more easily, have the peace of mind of trusting in your life, generating creativity and success, and open your heart and mind to better companions and friends in your life.

For in this new chapter of your life, you resourceful, even skillfully assume a more fullness to your heart and mind, your spirit, now magnetizing, each and anything, each and anyone, generating unstoppable and dramatic improvements, slowly, and skillfully, adept, with the skill of a master.

With each and every heartbeat, and each and every breath you take, not only does any and all of this happen, but forever and always, is now more relaxed and mighty you now know this to be true, now and forever, automatically your effective mind this time, works this out for you, while awake, while asleep, even while you dream, in the most powerful effective ways, known and unknown.

As other things arise, so too do you rise up, more easily and forever vanquishing challenges and shadows, more now than ever before, each and every day, each and every night, each and every moment, fearless and more trusting.

You become, you are and you remain, and new truth is awake inside of you, as you take your life more in stride, and from deepest recesses inside of you, as if a light shines down from above you on your all around you right now.

You have a sense, are given knowledge, it's all going to be okay, really just fine, better than ever.

Trusting in this forever and knowing it's truth and success.

Sports Performance Enhancement

Better Golf – Focus, Calm, Successful

You are calm, you are peaceful, you are relaxed, in fact relaxing ever deeper, into a brand new and better chapter of your life, unbeatably and unstoppably, feeling a shift in your energy and a rise in your inspiration.

Forever more calm, more successful, more easily able to remain in balance while staying focused, centered, and easily able to achieve success, driven forward by the energy of every past victory, triumph, breakthrough, inspiration, and success that you've ever had, almost as a feeling of blanket of that energy inspiring you and driving you forward unbeatably.

Any and all of this getting only easier and better each and every time you repeat this wonderfully enjoyable technique on your own.

Your correct response to any and all challenges presented to you from now over and finished previous chapters of your life, stepping forward into a brighter and better day in your life now forever, and sure of this, is to relax beyond any and all old former limits, into better moments of support, trusting in yourself, while relaxing and feeling an energetic a rush of vitality, strength, inspiration, a can-do spirit, and the ability to relax, and flow, dynamically breaking through, almost as if it's all happening on its own all around you.

In the past things may have been different, but you are certain that is now over, so whenever when you are around other people, you are instead sensing, feeling, and generating glowing and unlimited feelings of support from their presence around you, while being free forever of any issues about being viewed by them, as the more you are viewed, the more likely you are to succeed, shaking off all anxiety, becoming truly anxiety-free, sharply focused, and more easily able to break through unbeatably.

Free flowing while relaxing and focusing on your success, free of problems while steadfastly remaining challenge-oriented, you are now more easily able to stay focused and in the zone, achieving ultimate success, than any other time in your life, any and all of this only getting easier and better for you every day.

The way you play when you are alone is the way you will play in the presence of others, almost as if someone from deep, deep inside of you has reset a switch, a dial, a thermostat, or a computer of some kind, allowing you to play the game enjoyably like a professional - for what the pros know, you know, how they play, you play, how they think, you think, how they react, you react, how they move, you move, however they perform, especially while under pressure, is how you perform as well.

All you have ever seen, heard, or imagined about playing a better game, is now bubbling up to the surface to the unlimited power of your subconscious mind, breaking through here dynamically, unbeatably, and you are sure of this.

For all that you have learned is now more easily within your grasp and achieved, working in your favor, and whether you realize it or not, truly you have relaxed beyond former limits into a more free-flowing style of success.

Each and every practice swing is relaxed into, while being precise, smooth flowing and tension free.

Whenever you go to hit the ball, your body remains relaxed, almost as if memorizing this feeling you are now experiencing of total relaxation, relaxation being your correct response to any and all former challenge patterns, most especially whenever old challenge situations from previous now done chapters of your life may present themselves.

You are cool under fire and you cleverly remain tension-free.

Each and every swing, your body relaxed and flowing, free of over-thinking, each and every swing, flowing in perfect rhythm, and balance, professional skill, rhythm, and balance, as the ball proceeds forward from your body movements as an extension of your thoughts and your will, just as you desire and visualize.

Just like when at the practice range by yourself, you can always no matter where you are easily hit the ball long and straight just like the pros. For that is your way now, every swing and putt is your very best, doing even better, certain and sure.

Each and every swing, as smooth as any of your best practice swings have ever been.

Most especially whenever you have to take a short chip shot to the green, and just like your very best practice swings, you keep your head steady, you keep your eye on the ground, and you make the perfect swing.

Your days of second guessing and nervousness are now over, having blown away from you like a passing cloud now forgotten, instead and even better, you are focused, calm, clear, peaceful, and in the zone, even serene, watching the club and hitting the ball directly, moving your head just perfectly and sharing ultimate success that you now make your own.

You have done the work and you deserve the best all things, so here they are, flowing in proper rhythm and harmony, your mind cleverly adapting to this to make it work, while you are awake, while you are asleep, while you were dreaming, whether you are aware of this or not.

From now on, your days and nights are one of flowing and glowing success, completely rejuvenated and reinvented, not because I say so but because it is the nature of your own mind to achieve ultimate success here, and so it is and it remains as you are now cleverly and skillfully, adaptively reset, re-identified, and professionally rejuvenated.

In your imagination, let your mind wander back to a time when it was your best game.

So in the zone, so free flowing, so easily able, so breaking through - just like a golf outing with friends, even better.

Whether using any club or driver, you are now repeating this technique, in the zone each and every time you perform it. Every tee shot going down the middle, going up to the green, you are and you remain relaxed and carefree, free of over-thinking and free of being overly harsh to yourself.

You are in the moment, your body and movements, as well as the ball, going where you want it to be, relaxed and flowing.

You are working out loose ends and bringing it all together, each and every shot more perfect, summoning up free-flowing talent, all experiences leading you to success and greater understanding.

While the pressure is coming off, the fun is coming back, enjoying the fun and the love of the game, you perform at your own level, loving it so much, enjoying the game, loving the game and playing for fun, while enjoying yourself rather than pressuring yourself to play against others.

You play your own game for the fun of it all. Each and every time you play, you're playing as if alone.

The opinions, and competitive spirit of others against you means less and less. You know right now you are even better, and they actually inspire you to breakthrough and succeed further, as it is the fun and the love of the game that means more and more to you.

For when you believe in yourself you can do anything, but beyond belief there is faith, beyond faith there is simply knowing, and now you simply know all of this is getting easier and adaptively better for you, because you're playing any and all games focused upon your own talent, and you are liberating that talent out from heart and mind all around you, while playing as if alone on your own.

Each and every time you see a green golf course, the color green becomes a trigger signal for relaxation and relaxed concentration, achieving ultimate success.

Perfecting Your Golf Game

You take the pressure off. You relax into your swing. You relax into your game. You stop trying. You relax into it and everything just seems to flow.

When you are golfing and even when you are not golfing, your powerful and effective mind is now finding new and better ways to improve your game, in truly profound, amazing and powerful ways. You know from deep, deep inside, as a real and deep, powerful personal thought, the effective and potent fact that your love of the game shall always find a way.

Your love of your golf game is now expanding from deep, deep within you to find new, improved and better ways of playing and improving your game. Your love of the game is transcending all limits, flowing over around and through any and all past blockages, allowing your swing to flow, accurately, correctly, dynamically, precisely, as you relax into your game and improve in as yet unimagined ways.

The golf course is one of the most comfortable places in the world for you to be.

Your body and your muscles flow, you relax into this, you thrive, and you succeed, amazing and impressing everyone, most especially you.

The long clubs are now new friends, an accurate extension of you. They are allowing your very best energies to flow, all of your past moments of victory, breakthrough and inspired success are now allowing you to thrive and succeed.

As you relax deeper, you now imagine or wonder if you yet truly recognize and realize, that the inspiration of all of the pros, and all of their past moments of victory and inspired success are upon you now, allowing you to thrive and succeed, allowing you with their help to move on, unblocked, focused, willing, relaxed, totally able.

What they know you know. What they do, you do, so you do and it feels great, flowing, easy and powerful.

Now your swing and back-swing comfortably elongates *(or shortens)*. Everything for you now just seems to flow, flexible and flowing.

You are able to use the long tee, you get beyond the tee, relaxing into this, just flowing in body, emotion, mind and in spirit, moving on, you feel so very good now, confident, capable and able.

Frustration is leaving you now, like some sort of valve has been released, releasing the steam of past frustrations, allowing new and better satisfaction, gains, wins, pleasure, fulfillment, and happiness to flow in and be yours.

And all of your life works to support you in this, every thought, every feeling, every action, while you're awake, while you're asleep, even while you dream. You are effectively, flowingly, and precisely mending, healing and improving this.

You've begun a newer and better chapter of your life today. Re-identified, reinvented, released moving on, you feel and truly now know, getting only better and better, you are an unstoppable winner.

From deep, deep inside of your computer, a switch, dial, and a thermostat has been retained, reset, recalibrated to allow you and your golf game to work completely and unstoppably, with complete success, skillfully utilizing relaxation and sharper focus, as you are reset, retuned and rebalanced, while functioning optimally, forever and always a brand new chapter of your life, as your game just seems to flow through you naturally, heroically, sharp focus, in knowing and glowing confidence, or easily just in championship style.

For what the pros do you do, the pros know, you know, how they breathe, you breathe, how they move, you move, how they think, you think, how they feel, you feel, how they react, you react.

It's almost like in this brand new chapter of your life, their decades of knowledge are yours, their successful sense of pleasure is yours now.

Absolutely now, with each and every heartbeat and breath, you are more self-assured and serene, just right, so completely comfortable and so very much in your zone, and more easily able to function fluidly and in a flow, correctly achieving breakthrough success here, not because I say so, but because it is the nature of your own unstoppable mind to do this.

Safe and secure, calm and serene, you are, truly more certain of this each and every day and night, feeling inspired while you are awake, most especially while you're asleep, when you drift and float and dream. Your mind now always in the background working to achieve unbeatable, better success.

As you address the ball and take a practice swing, you keep your head down and make a good turn. But, now, in this brand new and better chapter of your life, when you hit the ball you always see the ball get hit, both body movements and eyesight like laser-beam precision as you stay down, relaxed and focused, now always free of ever lifting up. You always stay down, and of course the results are excellent.

Now reset and recalibrated, you always use your torso just properly and enough to skillfully complete your swing.

During the game whenever putting, in this new chapter of your life, which only thrives and succeeds, getting better, your focus and confidence are building and strong.

You are dynamic, even feeling fearless, and it feels like a rush of energy has strengthened you, focused you. You stay with the stroke, applying just the right pressure to your movement, holding the club gently, achieving unbeatable focus, skill, and results.

For the greater the challenge, the mightier are you are to rise up to deal with it.

When dealing with sand shots, you know the drill, while performing with amazing skill, impressing everyone, most especially yourself, as you hit about 2 inches behind the ball – and now in graceful flow you always do, you now and forever remain free of ever lifting up and sculling it, using just the right amount of swing to get the job done clearly, concisely, and effectively.

While having fun and feeling mighty, you always take the divot, looking forward to the challenge.

Free of devastating the ground, you connect and the ball seems to sail away exactly where it needs to be, as your focus is upon where it must land for maximum effect.

Every move of your body, every placement of your feet and legs and back and arms, every stroke that you take, every calibration that you make, every swing that you take, well adjusted.

Each and every club, the right choice, your clothing comfortable and supportive, easily free of distractions.

Just in the zone, in the moment, super and precise focus, precision and flowing movements, trusting in your skill, which is building, and building, and building, to achieve breakthrough ultimate success here, each and every thing working unbeatably in your favor.

Basketball Improvement

As you relax, your clever and adaptive subconscious mind is relaxing and working up numerous methods for life improvement, both known and unknown to you.

You are easily becoming more confident on the basketball court. The ball feels natural in your hands, a natural extension of your fingertips.

More confident in your abilities, decisions, and to basically feel that you truly belong on the court.

Intimidation-free of other players, focused and calm, for what inspires the pros, so inspires you. What they know, you know. What they do, you do.

How they move, you move and respond, fluidly and with expert timing, almost as if each and every time you repeat this exercise on your own, you are doing the equivalent of [12-14 years] worth of healing and improvement, worry free and powerful.

In fact, your heart, mind and all that is your very best, is now focused and easily generating success. You now play in a game as confidently and as aggressively and most importantly as well as you do in practice and when you are playing for fun.

You now relax even deeper, knowing this fact is automatically true.

All of this generates enjoyment and fun. You are relaxed, calm and cool, but at the same time play the game as aggressive as you always need to be.

Any and all nervousness, now left behind in past chapters of your life, finished, done over.

Free flowing, learning or succeeding, the pressure is off, you now flow onward, doing better and better.

Failure free, stress going and gone, each and every breath and heartbeat, more and more focused, calm, relaxed, flowing and capable, flowing and energetic, just getting any and all of this more effectively done with knowing, flowing movement and confidence, taking shots when you know the moment is right, and it is.

Mistake free, learning experience oriented, each and every time you play, run the ball, dribble, pass, shoot, more and more inspired, and moving beyond belief, just knowing. Moving and flowing like a pro, almost as if someone has forever reset, re-tuned or recalibrated you, adjusting a switch, a dial, a computer or a thermostat of some kind. Giving yourself a break, calm, focused, relaxed and inspired, failure free, learning, succeeding, and breaking though, a greater and greater player, more and more sure, self-assured and confident.

Knowing better and better is your legacy and best approach, heroically inspired, so unstoppable and determined and getting all and everything done that needs doing. Your mind relaxes and generates a true image of a successfully playing you, all of your best flowing moments now rising up to make you mighty, and you realize this now, or simply just know it as truth.

You opinion counts, you know who you are, getting it all done.

Each and every time, your perfection is evolving, craft fully and skillfully over time, so very in the moment, forever free of over thinking, smiling inside and outside now, as this gift of truth is now yours!

All and everything you do, learning and improvement now.

Each and every game, just doing better and better, trusting in life, you are doing well, focused and calm, you mind rehearses for each possibility, your body flows and enjoys the moments and flowing moments that are now yours.

Forgiven, released and healing, you thrive brilliantly, your mind working anything and everything out completely.

You prove to yourself only, you improve with each and every breath and heartbeat, learning and success is now yours.

You need to tune out the others, and you now tune into yourself, playing well for you!

You cut yourself a break, you choose to thrive or succeed, your energy balances, your very best restored, almost as if you are tapping all the energy you have to play, and channeling it just as it needs to be, all thoughts, actions and reactions, movements and attitudes, so amazingly self-supporting.

You end up playing, beautifully, better and better.

You are breathing smoothly, calm and serene, restoring you, and supporting you completely.

Mixed Martial Arts Enhancement

As you relax, deeper and further, you are relaxing beyond any and all former limits, into a place of relaxed focus, calmness, and concentration, and ultimate liberation of success.

Almost as if by relaxing right now, and as if every time you were repeating these enjoyable and highly effective relaxation techniques on your own, you are gaining the experience of sixteen years worth of additional training and skill, while cleverly and adaptively all around you to work with in your favor most especially whenever challenged.

For the greater the challenge, the greater your focus and more self assured you become and effectively remain. You are calm and peaceful and glowing, and knowing skill.

In this brand new and unstoppably beginning chapter of your life, you are turning and channeling the energy in previous and now forever done chapters of your life that once may have felt nervous, or uncomfortable, into the energy and strength, timing, pacing and skill, technique and adaptation, precise movements, as a single mindedness and focus of your intent all lead forward to victory and success that you sense and now make your own.

For the greater the energy in an environment around you, the more easily able you are to tap into that energy, make your own, seize it, internalize it, generate strength, boundless confidence, and effective skill, while utilizing it to your optimum advantage, even in surprisingly wonderful ways.

With each and every slow and steady breath that you take prior to a fight or a tournament or a test, each and every beat of your heart, every body rhythm, step and movement, is now sure, steady and strong, adapted, corrected and focused, precisely focused upon liberating and generating success.

It's almost as if, what the pros know, you know, what they do, you do, how they fight, you fight, how they move, you move, how they adapt, you adapt, how they pace, you pace, how they anticipate, you anticipate, how they float and flow, you too you.

Reversing any and all destructive energy, your success is liberated as potentials are fulfilled, knowing all of this from deep down inside, you are and steadfastly remain certain.

Any and all un-needed and unnecessary pressure is now off. You are failure free, liberating only ultimate success or learning.

For in this brand new and forever successful chapter of your life, you remain calm, cool, serene, energized - while redistributing energy to any of the places that support you, while easily and cleverly redirecting energy away from the places from now done and finished chapters of your life, that ever once stood and your way, not because I say so, but because it is in fact the nature of your own mind, body, emotions, and indelible spirit to do so.

Knowing this now, you are and you remain more certain and self-assured, calm and serene in your knowledge and strength, than ever before, of anything in your life.

You breathe as if inhaling and exhaling not only air, but calming and soothing inspiration, relaxation and focus through your navel as a source of light and healing, forever releasing and vanquishing imbalance and shadow, generating unbeatable performance skill and effective and inspired winning focus.

In your mind now, your mighty inner hero, the part of you that is so inspired and knows only complete success, is rising to the very top as a way to be, as a way to live, as a way to succeed and win.

This heroic you is unstoppable at anything you set your mind to.

All things now from the past that may have once felt overwhelming in any way, are now and forever effectively not only risen above, but energetically and in every other way, turned around, as the energy is now seized and utilized to work in your favor.

So very sure of this you are and you remain. Calm and serene, your inner hero liberates from inside of you, the [*master martial artist*] you have always been, as you now step forward into becoming forever a uniquely effective harmony and cadence with a new self-confidence and strength, becoming one with your inner winner.

Calm and serene, anxiety-free, you now are and forever remain, almost as if someone from deep, deep inside of you, has reset a switch, a dial, a thermostat, or a computer of some kind liberating from deep inside of you, right here and right now, a part of you that has already succeeded at some future point - becoming one with your success right here.

For the greater the challenge, the mightier and more effective you become. The bigger challenge and confrontation, the bigger the event - the calmer, the more skillful and centered, peaceful and serene, the more expert, the more sharp, and within the rhythm of the moment, you are and remain.

Even long before any event, every breath and heartbeat, while you are awake, while you were asleep, even while your dreaming, supportive and happy dreams of success, are all working expertly in your favor.

A new and more centered, effectively focused and championship level oriented you is now and forever surprisingly emerging.

Every little step forward brings forth greater and greater levels of dramatic success, sure of this forever you are and your certainly remain.

Whenever challenged by any joint or muscle in your body, during training or any competition, most especially your [*left knee*], you visualize, imagine, and can even feel, penetrating and healing golden-white life-force light restoring, healing, repairing, strengthening, even better than when brand new, complete flexibility, and restoration.

You now favor yourself and are doing all that it takes to rise up here and become effective and mighty. Your enjoyment and love of [*MMA/karate/etc*] is allowing you greater life-force, strength, and the ability to flourish in all things you've put your mind to.

It works well, and you work well, so naturally you will achieve satisfaction in all that you set your mind to. You allow your imagination and thoughts to support you in visualizing optimal outcomes that you seize and dynamically achieve. You step into the moment, you win, you are determined, succeeding and winning naturally.

You are strong, you are capable, you have great cardio endurance, and in this moment, you are more limitless and reset to the finest and highest optimum calibration.

You are and you remain steady, steadfast, effective, dynamic, and adaptive, self-assured, well prepared, focused, and embracing a future moment of victory, realizing highest potentials, so very easily liberated, amazing impressing everyone, most especially yourself.

Relationships

Greater Sexual Intimacy – Turned On Again – Women

And as you are relaxing, releasing, and feeling completely comfortable, all areas of restriction within your body, once blocked, or even knotted up at some point, are now being released, as you allow yourself to feel better about who you are, and rediscover feelings of intimacy between you and your [husband, lover, partner], naturally restoring itself, as if some major healing process is taking place, for truly and in fact, whether you realize it or not, perhaps you simply desire it, or in fact it truly is.

Feeling free, blockages released, you now release yourself and indeed rediscover feelings of oneness and intimacy [with your husband], allowing yourself to let go and to gain tremendous satisfaction.

In this place, in this new chapter, in this moment, only getting better and stronger and more adaptively effective, your body, your emotions, your mind, in fact all that you are, is being reconditioned, to a greater and greater level of intensity and turn on, build up, build up, and release, while release of past blockages frees you now completely, forgiven, healed, and as you are now and forever in a place of naturally occurring enjoyment, and better total passionate love, releasing all now done shadowy and forgiven emotional imbalances, now swept aside, you are now free and fulfilled, including any and all, both known and as yet unknown to you, guilt, fears, and blockages, now forever healed, forgiven and released, resetting and restoring you.

You now know this to be true, not because I say so, but because it is in fact a reality for you, a forgiven choice, the correct decision you have made, absolutely feeling released, relaxed and calm, and more unrestricted, energies redirected, healthy, whole, healed, you now truly know this as truth, while you are awake, when you are sleep, even while you dream, your mind now free and working things out, forever unblocked and released, remaining unblocked, and focused, easily able, to relax your way, through previous restricted barriers.

Your correct response, to any and all of this, reacting by slower and comfortable easy breathing, and allowing your breath to take its own natural course, to release, and like a flower, open you up to something more enjoyable and fulfilling, each and every little step meaning a lot, each and every little step, moving forward on your journey, breaking through here unbeatably, feeling serene and peaceful, achieving all that you wish to naturally, released, forgiven and open.

Although feelings from past chapters of your life may have taken a short vacation or a temporary hiatus, really truly and now and forever done, right now on this brand new chapter, it is almost as if someone from deep, deep inside of you, has reset a switch, a dial, a thermostat, or some kind of a computer, actively reviving and reactivating, energizing, healing, and rejuvenating you in all the ways should express your love, fulfillment, building and building ecstasy and intimacy [with your husband], to a place of greater heights, and a place of greater youth, and a place of greater excitement, and the place of greater enjoyment. You have just now, in fact, let go, while releasing yourself to experience those correct and right feelings again.

It just feels great to be so certain that you have released any and all imbalance, any and all doubt or fear, serene and anxiety-free, comfortable within your own skin and with your own building passionate sexual desire, as any and all of your very best intimacy thoughts, sexual feelings, sexual fantasies, even though ones you've never shared with anybody, that turn you on the most, are now rising to the top freeing you once and for all, judgment free, in a moment, experiencing life as it was meant to be for you, breaking through barrier-free right here and now.

It is natural, it is okay to be fine being just who you are, fully a woman now, the energy is there and building and building, vital energies and blood flow now directed and restored.

Your passionate desire to break through has guided you, all thoughts and feelings. When it comes to [your husband], more easily turned-on, physical sensations, just the way you like them, passionate thoughts, desires and feelings, just the way they ought to be, and a more balanced and enhanced set of nerve endings and even hornier and passionate response, flowing through your system.

The power of your mind and your spirit, every thought and feeling, every action and reaction, reset, rejuvenated, actually recalibrated, intensified, breaking you through here more easily, for in your mind you now know, from foundational places deepest inside of you, that you are and you remain more interested, struggle-free and free of trying, relaxed, turned on, tingly, easily enhanced desire, imagination, translating into joyous intimacy, love.

Building up and release, imagination relaxed, wide open and ready, and more stimulating with every thought and feeling, every breath and heartbeat, and focused, more easily successful, embracing any and all aspects of yourself, your femininity, and your womanliness, wide open each and every time, greater intimacy, to generate greater levels of intimacy, relaxed, calm and determined, one building on the next to break you through here unbeatably.

Like relaxing and enjoying sexuality and sexual actions as well as sensations to achieve orgasm, now better than ever before. Feeling more attraction and being more attractive yourself, you are now better and more easily building passion, are now having more sensual and wandering sexual imagination, thoughts and feelings, even fantasies, that build greater enjoyment attraction, and intimacy from deep inside of you each and every day.

Your femininity and ability to be a sexy woman, your body just right, attractive to you and to [your husband], just now feeling better and more okay about yourself and in every moment, you know, you believe you think, 'it's okay to be me and all that I am.' Here now enjoying each sexual moment more and more.

Whenever engaged sexually and intimately with [your husband] more easily aroused and stimulated in just the way should like it best enjoying yourself while fulfilling yourself sexually while bringing pleasure to both of you.

Seduction and passionate intimacy, leads to more powerful and more fulfilling buildup and release. More satisfied and fulfilled by intimacy and more easy sexual intimacy, as you are, and you remain. You've worked it out and so it is, relaxing, now enjoyable, you just doing better and better.

Any touch, your thoughts, your heart, your skin, your body, your breasts, nipples, vulva, clitoris, or anyplace you have found pleasurable, now restored, and released, effective, more loving, more enjoyable, more intimate, hot and exiting you, more and more, more and more, more and more.

Feeling wonderful and better and better, in just the very best ways you enjoy it most, and in the ways that are best for you and [your man] to enjoy the best, released and pleasured, at your very best.

Any and all extras, working in your favor, romantic moments, kissing, holding each other, acts and actions of intimacy, even hand-holding, generate the embrace and sense of the oneness of lovers' energy and passionate desire.

Any sort of sexual stimulation, or romantic, emotional or mental sexual stimulation, all easily and effectively achieve maximum benefit, right then from deep within you, any touch, more happy, sexy, pleasurable and tingly between you and [your man], activating and achieving powerful and fulfilling romantic enhancement.

Leading you to feel, know, sense and experience a reliving of your real life memory of the feelings that precisely and correctly, potently and powerfully lead to more enjoyable building and building sexual stimulation in whatever ways the two of you more fulfillingly and well deservedly build, as your body and mind truly reconditioned, now easily relax down the path leading to more profoundly fulfilling and even full body orgasms, each and every moment enhancing the previous moment.

Relaxed and frustration free, it be comes better, and more intimate generating loving oneness between the two of you.

Feel the joy and the intimacy now yours, happy and delighted inside and out, free at long last, it feels great to be so free. Confident and free, you have broken through.

One thing excitedly builds upon the next, the sensations of your skin, in perfect concert with your sexual sensations and organs, things working right, better and better than right, your passionate desire and love, the oneness both of you share, all build to a more fulfilling and loving experience, a joining of heart and mind, bliss, because it feels right and wonderful, it is right and wonderful, released and deserved, having now, in this unstoppable new chapter of your life, calmly gotten out of your own way, and so you have.

As it was when you were younger, more and more excitement and enhanced.

You now more interested in achieving oneness and fulfillment, appropriately sensitive, sensations and feelings, tingling, building and building pleasurable feelings, redirected blood flow budding desire, and a passionate feeling activated from your mind, into the wanting and desired fulfillment.

Turing on, you orgasm building and flourishing, more easily and powerfully, comfortably, free of ever trying, build and release, so it just happens and comes, you relax and the feeling is increased and more right, eight to fifteen times better, yes, sensitivity just the way you like it, things now more and more just right, sensitive in just the way you love it and have always enjoyed it best, simply and really, now even more so.

Your thoughts, feelings, actions, and reactions, all corrected and in concert, building and building a greater closeness and oneness with your pleasure, relationship, ecstasy, sexuality, release, fulfillment, [husband] and sexual excitement and orgasmic release.

Experiencing sexual turn-ons together, secret intimacies, shared thoughts, all okay now, and better, blood flow and bodily fluids building there, all building great success and passion, fulfilling deep, deep, passion, each fantasy, thought, your attraction to him, and with him, fulfilling you both, as if 19 again, all those and better and better feelings and sensations return, although now even better and more fulfilling.

As you really enjoy sex again and sex with [your husband] becomes an event, looked forward to with freeing anticipation, and fun. Finding now new and better things within that, achieving greater love, passion, and more fulfilling sexual climax than ever before.

Finding the love that you have in your heart is easily translated now in this new chapter of your life, and you more sexual expressive and enjoyable. Hotter, wetter, more excited and better.

All of this relaxation response actually allows you to bring forth into your life right now in this moment, feelings and experiences of oneness intimacy, pleasure and release, the feeling and well-deserved sexual pleasure, orgasm and intimacy.

You deserve this, you create this, you relax and flow beyond barriers, the barriers are now dissolved, you now certain, sure, and serene, more passionate and loving, in a brand new chapter of your life certainly and forever, absolutely certain and surely your desire activating more than enough energy that transforms you into this, or liberate you as needed to be what you always have been.

As you desire for intimacy and oneness with [your husband] just seems to build and build easily from the automatic part of your mind each and every day and night.

You deserve this, you reactivated, it's achieved, powerfully and refreshingly as you are now restored and released. A new and more improved woman, now is who you are.

Wandering back in your imagination, go back to a time and see yourself, picture yourself, notice, imagine, or even know yourself, at the age of [nineteen.]

And in this moment allow that image of yourself, that sense, that feeling, more excitable and more pleasure achieving and fulfilling you, to become one with you. What she feels and experiences, you know you'll experience, her energy, now yours, her ability to express and enjoy sex, oneness, pleasure, and orgasms, yours.

All energies, all nerve endings, all blood flow, all passion, all desire, all intimacy, get better and more fulfilling, and you now, wiser, even better, based on experience, released, successfully, allows you to bring forth an upgraded even better and improved version of a more sensual you, all of this effectively instilled and empowered by her and you as you, as never before.

You now know, your powerful and dynamic subconscious mind working this out in ways beneficial and breakthrough to you, in ways both known and unknown to you, sharing an increasing sexual relationship, satisfaction and intimacy and more joy, pleasure, as a better way with the [man] you love, sharing that love, experiencing greater love, and sexual passion, release, and fulfillment.

Forgiving/ Moving Beyond Past Abuse

You are, as of this time, forever finished with sorrow and old memories as a way of life.

In this moment, you are determined to feel good and happy about your life, your world and your past.

You are already forgiving, releasing and powerfully moving beyond any and all upset, in dynamic ways, forgiving them and more especially, yourself and your attachment, to anything disturbing.

For in this moment, as you relax deeper and further, you are putting any and all past burdens down, down right now, down for good, down forever.

Your powerful correct response to any and all old sorrow or upsets, disturbing memories and suffering, is to relax and forgive your way out of those moments.

So in this moment of profound and deep relaxation, you have finally and even dynamically, truly decided to know that all of these things, have in fact polished you, for not only have you decided to see those things as things you not only powerfully survived, but each and every circumstance and event has truly and forever polished you.

You actually feel as if an unstoppable surge of energy, the energy of every past victory, triumph, breakthrough, and success you've ever felt, had or even imagined, is upon you now, allowing you to thrive and succeed beyond any and all past blockage, releasing powerfully, as never before.

So you'll always decide to flow beyond, or to succeed, and it feels great.

I wonder if you even yet realize how easy this is going to be for you as you relax, rise above your past easily and triumphantly.

For in this moment, and in all and any future moments, only getting more powerful, easy and successful, you are liberated free and strong.

You easily move on with your life and improve the years you have ahead.

As you relax deeper and further, further and deeper, from deepest recesses of your mind, you begin to release, relax, and relieve yourself, generating complete and total relief for yourself, in the most potent and powerful ways possible.

Your mind is now absolutely determined, as well as all of the rest of you, and is becoming forever more determined, to relinquish, and relieve yourself, of any and all unresolved, unreleased, uncomfortable, even upsetting, emotions feeling or thoughts and habits, both known and unknown to you, releasing them completely and absolutely, in ways both known and unknown to you, to your complete maximum benefit, and ultimate release and relief.

You begin to jettison the cargo of unresolved emotions, resolving them, and releasing them, as so much more on each and every breath, on each and every heartbeat, as with every movement of your body, you are letting them go, as you have now more completely than ever before, decided to benefit yourself and to relieve yourself, burden free, of things that no longer serving and supporting you to maximum benefit.

You have simply chosen to forgive, release, relent, let go of and move away from, each and every thought, feeling, emotion, memory, experience, both real and imagined, that have ever stood in your way and as by releasing them, support yourself, to maximum success, and ultimate breakthrough, free at long last, more now than ever before. You simply choose a life of learning with less discomfort, processing discomfort and letting it go.

Generating comfort more completely, with each and every breath and heartbeat, every day, every night, every moment, this becomes easier, more productive, and better for you.

Your imagination wonders, as a new thought arises, *I choose to process life's lessons and my experiences in more self-supporting and self-loving ways.*

You now choose to embrace the energy of healing, while healing, completely releasing, letting go of and totally forgiving any and all past traumas, generating a life supporting and nurturing blanket of forgiveness and loving energy to yourself.

For the mightier than challenge once was in past moments of your life, the mightier you are able now to rise up, release and forget that, trauma free, whole and healthy, restored and heroically motivated to break through here and succeed.

This is the option you choose, it is your only option, usual way now, and so it is in forever remains.

All discomfort releases and relieves itself from you in ways most appropriate, and even in surprisingly effective amazing ways.

Even your dreams support and relax you, so even at night you relax and unwind, and even now realize you are in a new chapter of your life now, treating yourself better, vanquishing the discomfort of the past, as it no longer serves you, you've thrown it completely and forever aside, cast it overboard, as you now know it washes away, far, far away from you.

It feels good to be so relaxed and relieved, so at night when you sleep, your dreams calm you down, your mind relaxes, you have put your life up on a shelf, at night, all through the night, able to rest peacefully and sleep, regenerating, restoring, taking better care of yourself, as this begins to happen on its own automatically, mind, relaxed, clear and free, forgiven and healing, whole, healed, doing better and better, relieved.

It's becoming easier and better for you to accomplish this, as you are now in a Divinely guided place of restoration and healing, all healing you seek, generated from the deepest recesses inside of you, now takes place as a cascade of healing, unstoppable and forever.

You embrace the rest of your life, as an internal flow, and a place of polished, unbridled success.

It is almost as if you have been restored, all the emotional and balance, upset, and trauma from now on vanquished, and done, because your mind is automatically working this out, in ways so pleasing, so happy, so calming, so relieving, so releasing, so precise, so perfect, so right, so self-loving, so much more noticeably healthy, for you, than ever before, as you relax beyond former limits.

Just relax and flow, to the place you need to be most.

So whether it's sleep, or inspired thoughts of a lighter, healthier than a better you, all of it works in concert to break you through.

Break Up Survival -- Moving On for Women

Your greatest desire is to be free and in a new chapter of your life, and so you are, truly living this desire into reality. And so you now know you are free of needing in any way. The greatest need to take care of yourself and your son lovingly, and the very best of ways. Having done the equivalent of [7, 16, 22] years of healing, release, and self-love. all of this making sense to you in the deepest and most foundationally beneficial of ways.

The best way to control anything, is to relax and flow, releasing any and all concept of control. So that, in fact, is what you begin to do.

You relax, you trust, you come from a better and more vital place, almost as if from the deep, deep inside of you, someone has reset a switch, the dial, a thermostat, or a computer of some kind, once and for all, certainly and most assuredly, having reset and recalibrated you into a brand new and better self loving chapter of your life.

Things you once tried to change, become more dramatically and more substantially less important, as more and more your life is working more in your favor, every thought, more beneficial and supportive, every feeling, released and replaced by better feelings of adequacy and self-support, every action taken by you working decisively in your favor in self-supporting ways only.

You are free of needing always to depend on another, depending instead on the parts of yourself with your inner wisdom and strength, now active and released into the world around you and into your life.

Every reaction to anything in your world, now more substantially healthy, life-giving and emotionally strengthening and stabilizing to you [and to your child], in the most beneficial of ways, not because I say so, but because it is the nature of your mind to do this, and therefore, so it is, and so remains forever.

You are learning, having learning experiences, failure-free, free of mistakes, choosing to either only learn or succeeded in your life, refreshed in heart and mind, substantially stronger and better, clearer, more adaptive, more easily able to transcend, putting the past into the past.

Now free and released, more determined to achieve this dramatically and in the most potent and effective ways, that stabilize and substantially reinforce and support you, and all that is your life, and all of those you truly love, [like your son, as his mother,] most especially a condition that loving and supporting yourself, and the very best of ways, emotionally, mentally, physically even spiritually.

For there you are, and there you are for yourself, more loving and self-supportive, than ever before.

As you relax deeper and further, you recognize and embrace a new truth, that only you can be there for yourself, and all you can change from within you.

Things once causing friction and discomfort, now cleverly worked out, working out and adaptably released, clearing the way and allowing room self-support, relaxation, release, and transcendence, as all things once found to be a hindrance, are now forever released, as if less and less important to you, as if it happening decades ago, almost as if cloudy in memory and feeling, practically forgotten and completely unimportant, as it feels good to be so comfortable, happy and free, truly wanting and enjoying the experience, of being free.

You know -- Ahhh, free at long last!

You pick your spots, you know which challenges to take on with varying degrees of challenge, and releasing anything and everything futile from the past, having been polished by it and having grown up so much more than those experiences now forever released and done.

Each and every day, each and every night, each and every breath, each and every heartbeat, and experience of you learn how to love yourself better and better.

Feeling this now, your heart lights up with self-love, your mind and emotions restore balance, as you are and you remain, treating yourself like someone you love, every thought, every feeling, every action and reaction, leading into the masterpiece of a better life you deserve, generating all of this recreates yourself.

You now, once and for all, forever and always, this is true.

I wonder if you even yet realize how truly easy this is going to be for you, or simply in this moment - you have succeeded, heroically stepping forward, and becoming one with this new and improved you, having truly moved on.

Your ever-increasing love for yourself, and self respect, from a force and deep, deep inside of you has now been activated to achieve any and all of this, pushing away from yourself things that are all once were self destructive.

You are restored, self supporting and loving, just like a Phoenix rising from its own ashes.

Any and all actions you generate allow you to now feel reborn into a new chapter of your life, benefit from the experience, as you are now and cleverly remain free at long last, you now know this to be true.

For when you learn to love yourself, the only love you will experience is one that is unconditional with yourself and eventually with someone new.
Any and all of this leads you to become stronger energetically and mentally.

You deserve to feel joyful, you remember that sense and feeling and therefore you recreated immeasurably, becoming a masterpiece of joy!!

YOU DESERVE to feel good and be deeply happy, and so you cleverly create this, good and deeply happy you are and you remain, adaptive enough to make this happen.

Releasing and letting go of the discomfort that once was inside of you.

It's released as you let it out.

There is only room for joy, love, and rising above all challenges, and the most dynamic of ways, throughout all that is your mind and body.

You find comfort within yourself, you are all that you need, you give yourself what is unique.

You need you, and you become an endless reservoir of love, and support, inspiration caring for yourself, free of expectations of others, you are taking so much better care of yourself right now.

Any and all of this generates a greater capacity for deepest and most complete, well-deserved, mental stability and compassion within yourself, free of sympathy, effectively releasing worry, you dynamically create trust, trusting in life, worries are trivial, activating your inner hero, you rise up and succeed mightily.

Being filled up with love inside yourself, your greatest need is to enrich and enlighten yourself, while releasing stress, truly calmer and better, generating love, and experiencing a better life.

Doing everything and anything and honestly takes to succeed.

Dynamically now and forever you do your very best, to rise up beyond limiting circumstances, and in every moment seek to be the best that you can be in each and every circumstance for the greater the challenge, the more loving, adaptive, honest and clever you become, as you generate breakthrough and healing.

Being filled up with love inside yourself, there is no need for anyone else, you are enough and doing better and better, in ways yet unimagined, cleverly, fulfilled and lovingly.

Released, relaxed and restored, you now knowing, you are doing better and better.

Female Fertility Extra

As you relax, float, drift and dream, you always knew and now powerfully and forever know, your desire to get pregnant comes to fruition in this brand new, better and unstoppable chapter of your life.

Gone automatically are the blockages and hindrances of the past, feeling and now knowing you are and you remain forever free, in ways both known and unknown to you.

You're embraced by a higher light, which is unstoppably balancing and restoring you, in a wave of unconditional love and truth and deepest forgiveness release of any and all things, even people, [most especially your mother, grandmother and mother-in-law].

Ahhhh, feeling incredibly better and better now, rising up mightily, things that once blocked your way, are now and forever released into the past, almost as if it were years ago, even a million years ago.

You now believe, but beyond belief there is faith, beyond faith, really, you now simply know, you have all the time you need, relaxing deeply and truly all over, knowing from deepest and most sincere places inside, more now than ever before, that it will happen.

Released, reinvented, and rejuvenated, you profoundly see yourself as fertile.

You now truly see and know your body especially your wonderfully supportive and healthily functioning internal organs are healthy, whole, balanced, restored; complete, beautiful and cooperative.

On each and every breath and heartbeat, every action and reaction, you now truly know that you can make a healthy baby.

Beer & Alcohol

Alcohol Free

You may have been drinking for [20] years, or since you were [17], but you now know that's now done, you've moved on, you've grown up just a little bit more, that it's in the past.

Your present and future are now available free, taking better care of yourself, as you now know better about who you are, loving and trusting in yourself.
For the greater the challenge, the mightier you become. You're confident, calm, and serene, knowing who you are, comfortable in all situations, most especially social situations.

Even when you see another person drinking, you are more alcohol free, choosing something better for yourself, something healthy and good for you, you're taking better and more loving care of yourself, so inspired an unbeatable, you are now unstoppable for success through any and all of this.
Your greatest wish was to become and forever remain alcohol free, and in this moment, you have made that choice. It has now been for always and forever, almost like you never drank again after that day.

You more easily and cleverly stick to the idea of creating a more problem free life, this time doing better and smarter things, trusting in your life, doing smart healthy things now even better and instead.

Your days of getting drunk, were but a bump in the road, and you now move further away from that place every day and every night.

You're determined to take better care of yourself for your family and those that you love, for the greater the love, the more determined you become, truly you become, the better you feel, taking the very best care of yourself. You have chosen to become and forever remain free of hard alcohol, any and all alcohol, taste and smell, even light beer, so very disgusting.

You remain alcohol free, calm and anxiety-free, instead choosing to feel and remember how to feel, peaceful, serene, gentle to yourself, taking better care of yourself.
Feeling more confidence, you choose to be comfortable, realizing that you are enough, and people like you for who you are, taking better care of yourself, drink healthy alcohol free, most especially when challenged in highly social situations, like parties or boring conversations, you take a greater interest in people and in your life.

For whatever any famous person or celebrity can do, you now make your own and do so as well, alcohol free. The feel of an alcoholic drink in your hand or up to your mouth so very uncomfortable, just plain wrong, not healthy. You are doing better, each and every day and night, easier and better as your results improve.

Free of Drinking Beer and Alcohol

In this moment of deep relaxation, your mind has made a new association, to rise up and become mighty, heroic, becoming slightly more of an adult, easily able to be a child, however putting aside the things of childhood, and the things that once forever stood in your way, you are now always and forever free from.

Just as growing up from your childhood into adulthood has spurred you forward into new things, your tastes have improved, become more refined, have change in your favor, for example, various treats as a child, not as appealing as often, nor as much, so now, neither is beer or alcohol.

More attractive and even better liked, free of drinking beer, admired, more than ever before.

In this moment of deep and inspirational relaxation, you choose to treat yourself better, in ways more healthy, mightier, and to relieve yourself of the burden of alcohol consumption.

No longer seen as an old friend, now better seen as a destructive and deadly product, something you must remove from your life and all costs.

And now it is gone, you have made the right choice, the wise choice, acting in your favor, while fulfilling your greatest moments, stepping forward into your life, more stress-free, more self actualized, loving yourself better than to ever backslide ever again, into that miserable place that stands in the way of your health.

Relieving any negative reputations about yourself, in fact now you, a shining example to each and every woman and man who beholds you, as a person who is heroic, has reached and risen up, has become mighty, and is now free of the burdens of self destruction like alcohol and beer.

On each and every breath and each and every heartbeat anything and everything that ever once caused you to drink, now reversed to keep you drinking healthy liquids, beer and alcohol free.

Any and all of this becoming easier for you, not because I say so, but because of your decision of putting your foot down, and saying no to beer and alcohol, and so it is and so would remain forever.

It's almost as if someone from deep, deep inside of you has reset a switch, a dial, a thermostat of some kind, that allows you to break through here, while fulfilling yourself, filing you with self esteem and self confidence.

To know who you are, is simply OK. You are enough, and so you are and so it is and so it becomes.

Free of beer, free of alcohol, you now free, the burden off your back, at long last.

Ahhhhh, it feels so great to be so free.

New habits for health and self actualization begin now, on each and every breath and heartbeat, you now more firmly pulled into the light of healing, as a brighter, healthier, more playful, more upbeat you begins right now, restoring your health, your reputation, and a balance in your life that lasts forever.

You become forceful and true to yourself, remaining free of alcohol and beer, as you know that even just a little tiny bit is poisonous to you.

You are taking better care of yourself, most especially whenever challenged, most especially when in social situations. When in the past you said yes, now you say no.

Whether it's a party or a wedding, any social situation, while feeling comfortable and relaxed, and more happy about who you are, seeing something of yourself and everyone you meet, easily able to converse and relate yourself to the world around you.

You are enough, you are self loving, ensuring that you are loved and rejuvenated and reconditioned, inside and out.

Whether at work, or ay home, on the phone, anywhere, any and all of this is becoming easier, almost like with each and every breath you take, and each and every beat of your heart, you have moved forward five, eight, fourteen years into the future, again and again, so much more and more free of these issues.

You are now in your own words and thoughts, feelings, inspirations and ideas, powerfully and forever willing to do whatever it takes to become and remain healthy.

You effectively work on your self-esteem, as you now and trust more of yourself, you gain and win confidence, feeling more comfortable with yourself, and with every person you meet.

As you relax, so inspired, so at one with your life and the world and the universe, you somehow notice, imagine, picture, or simply just know, now you are and remain comfortable with people, feeling comfortable about them as well as yourself.

You begin to release these issues in your life that stand in your way, becoming one with the universe and all people in it.

You even find reasons or perhaps excuses to become more at one with the wonderful life in the world around you, alcohol free, beer free .

The days of lying to yourself are over, you are ready to take on your own inner power, activating highest inner light, which brings inner and outer wisdom while releasing everything and anything that no longer serves you, most especially alcohol and beer.

Beer and Alcohol Extras

Each and every time you are with friends, you are so much better off, much more at ease, much more at home in your own skin, much move relaxed, alive, happy, funny, animated, a better friend to yourself and others, a good talker and a better listener free of drinking beer and being true to yourself and loving yourself.

You have the confidence to know better, being done with it and moving forward, forgiven, healed, healthier, and better off, sober, and living better, driving safely, true to yourself and those you love most, most especially loving yourself more and better off.

Newer and better responses to stress and stress relief begin to emerge, and take better care of you.

Your correct response to any and all stress is to take slow and steadying deep and soothing breaths and relax all over, calm down.

Drinking water brings support and relief.

Deep breathing, stress flowing all around you, past you and beyond.

Whether stressed or bored, or feeling any kind of emotion, you've grown up, moved on and are simply done and doing better for yourself, your life, your marriage, those you love, those who love you.

New and better habits, new and better friends, almost divinely inspired, or simply just unstoppable, free of drinking beer and doing better for yourself, in ways both known or unknown to you.

Each and every day and night, a shining example of what it's like to have moved on, the truth is here, true and honest with yourself, honestly losing the taste of alcohol for better tasting and life giving liquids, water, juice.

Good times, great times, better times, better you, better life, this gift is yours, a new chapter of your life, more enjoyable, better, less stress, more complete, in ways both known and unknown to you, whether alone or with others, having outgrown the past, your very best rising to the top, in this new and unbeatable chapter of your life, all working out automatically, now is your unstoppable time to thrive.

Session Optimizing Statements (SOS)

1-89, covering a variety of subjects

Session Optimizing Suggestions

SOS 1: You will only receive powerful and precise, highly effective and beneficial improvement in the most correct, potent, extremely effective, powerfully correct and fluidly adaptive ways from this.

You are easily going into this wonderful relaxation state faster, deeper, stronger and better, with more limitless results in more unlimited dynamic ways every time you repeat this extremely enjoyable, wonderful, dynamic, highly effective and precise exercise.

SOS 2: The whole world works to support you in all of this, every sound, every noise that you hear from outside, including sirens, car horns and car alarms, (barking dogs, etc.) each and every time you hear them instantly reinforce all of this.

Even ringing telephones, every time you hear them are instantly reinforcing all of this, most especially your freedom and liberation from ... *(e.g. smoking, overeating, gaining weight, your old habit, your fear, your phobia, etc.)*

SOS 3: In fact, you feel like you've got the whole world in the palm of your hand. You are a winner. An unstoppable force of life improvement from deep within you has been forever activated. Your awareness grows, your life expands, you are both now and forever free and you truly know it.

SOS 4: And your self-confidence, self-esteem and inner strength will immediately increase. You will detach completely from all conflicts, frictions and disharmonies, feeling forever free. You are empowered, successful and liberated.

With every breath that you take, with each and every beat of your heart, your strength and dynamic empowerment increases, every suggestion and every beneficial solution and strategy, even adaptation you mind resolves, instantly activate, amazing and impressing everyone, especially even you!

SOS 5: You begin to take even better care of yourself, re-identifying and re-defining yourself as a new happier, energetic and lighter hearted person, by allowing newer and more empowered thoughts and inspired feelings of success, healing, wellness, breakthrough and health, each and every day to profoundly build within you like a giant reservoir of limitless energy and you allow yourself to bring forth the true reality, that you are whole, calm, comfortable, successful, lighter, better and complete.

SOS 6: Your desire to succeed becomes a passion, your passionate desire becomes a truly committed unstoppable force, each and every day and night, you overwhelmingly succeed in truly inspired, effective, creative, amazing and successful ways, relaxing into a brand new better chapter of your life, winning in the most profound ways! You have no idea how easy this is going to be for you.

SOS 7: With each and every breath you take, you are powerfully liberating the feelings, energy and sensations associated with these following thoughts, ideas and concepts into a vital and profoundly true reconditioning and redefinition of who you are, where you live from, how you respond and whom you grow forever to be into your life. You are feeling wonderful and forever improving by becoming *(name the feelings, actions and reactions you wish to instill).*

SOS 8: *(While they are deeply hypnotized)* Nod your head for me because you now and forever truly know, that you've forever relaxed your way into a brand new and better chapter of your life and really know that all of this is true. *(wait for their nod and then continue).*

SOS 8 A: *(While they are deeply hypnotized)* Nod your head for me because you know that this is true. *(wait for their nod and then continue).*

SOS 9: You trust in and truly know this fact: Each and every moment of your life is improving and that things get better and more surprisingly and astoundingly wonderful for you in each and every way.

SOS 10: You are feeling a new, correct, true and profound sense of support from your life, urging you ever onward into a lifetime of clever success.

SOS 11: It might really even seem like it's been at least 4, 12 or 16 years since you last (*smoked a cigarette, overate, felt stressed, etc.*), it's just so long ago, so forever ago, so far away from you, so far away your mind, your emotions, your habits and your life right now. In amazingly powerful, highly effective and important ways, you are truly liberated, cleansed, safe and forever free.

SOS 12: Just as you've always done, you are doing everything you've put your mind to, to get the job done, the most efficient of ways, most especially. . .(*quitting smoking forever, losing weight, reducing stress, etc*).

SOS 13: By becoming ever increasingly determined to feel good, you are surely feeling fine, wonderful and fantastic. So with each and every beat of your heart and with each and every breath that you take, you are relaxing deeper and further and your whole life forever improves.

SOS 14: It's almost like you are jumping over the years back to a time when you were (XX, 12) years old, and only this time, you are making powerful and forever commitment to yourself, so that even when you were (XX, 13), you were, remained and forever are (*smoke free, cigarette free, . . . or . . . . lighter, thinner, healthier, better, more active . . . or calm, balanced, rising above and beyond any and all stress, etc*), for then, for now, forever and for always, living better, happier and more successfully in the very best and well deserved of ways.

SOS 15: You will always remember to breathe deep and steady powerful soothing, breath; a calming, centering, stilling, harmonizing and balancing breath, and by doing so, you are easily overcoming any and all fear, doubt, worry and panic.

That which once overwhelmed you, is now both easily and forever powerfully overwhelmed by you and the power of your breath, as you leave all fear, panic, and discomfort, far, far behind you forever. All fear, doubt and panic are now and forever forgiven, released, healed and vanquished.

SOS 16: Now that you are proud of yourself and sure of yourself, you are amazingly unstoppable at all of this, feeling forever proud of yourself and permanently improved, taking your life back, truly getting amazingly successful, fluidly adaptive and precisely effective results from this highly proficient and enjoyable experience, going into this deeper, faster and even better results, every time you repeat this exercise.

SOS 17: You are easily free of anyone throwing you off track by saying any words or even expressing any feelings, thoughts or actions that might stand in your way here. You are in fact feeling mighty and you are easily rising above and masterfully transcending any and all old limits, now in this brand new chapter of your life.

SOS 18: The truest and most real point of view that matters to you is your own. In the long run, the opinions of others are just that, just points of view, to be learned from, embraced or even to be just put aside.

You put aside everything and anything that interferes with your ever-growing success, whether it's opinions of others, stress, emotional feelings, mental patterns or even old blockages most especially any and all of the things that once caused you discomfort or distress. You are becoming clearer, sharper, better, more fluid and adaptive, more flexible and unstoppably successful.

SOS 19: Now that you are learning to truly appreciate yourself, you can do anything you've now and forever, set your unstoppable and effectively adaptive mind toward. Each and every thing you do and on each and every breath and on each and every heartbeat, you are cleverly adapting and succeeding at this as never before!

SOS 20: You have now made up your powerful, adaptive, highly effective mind, which is only now working in your favor, getting stronger, better and more effective at reducing and eliminating any and all disruptive thoughts, feelings, actions and reactions, that once caused you to *(name behavior)*, choosing now instead to deep breathe, to calm down and to thrive and succeed forever in their place.

You are finding newer and better, more completely adaptive, fluid, skillful and eminently successful ways of reducing and even eliminating any and all old behaviors that once blocked you or stood in the way of your success now in favor of a newer and better well deserved life you now powerfully, effectively and adaptively create.

SOS 21: Each and every beat of your heart and each and every breath that you take, is easily reinforcing all of this in the most powerful and potently adaptive effective ways. You are glowing on the inside with all of the limitless energy of inspired success.

SOS 22: It's time to clean up your life, so you are and you are succeeding powerfully, adaptively, surely and with ever growing, more determined, creatively inspired, limitless success.

SOS 23: In your past, one of your urges may have been *to (name behavior: smoke, overeat, etc)*. However now and forever, your greatest urge, an unstoppable urge that's building up to being at least 178 times greater, growing ever stronger is to remain healthy safe and free *(name desired result: smoke free, cigarette free, etc)*.

SOS 24: Your greatest and most overwhelming craving is to become and forever remain healthy, happy free and safe, extending your life in ways that work for you best.

SOS 25: Regardless of any and all past challenges, you truly and foundationally know right now, in the long run, a better day will surely dawn. That dawn begins right now, illuminating your life, going on forever, freeing you and healing you, making your life the very best it can be, as you feel content and smile happily from, deep, deep inside.

SOS 26: It has been said, the one thing we never get back in life it time, every moment wasted on trivia, disharmony, imbalance and minutia, is a wasted moment of our most valuable asset, ourselves, our life, and our life-force.

You are easily enjoying and employing all of your very best energies, to make the most of every well deserved and well feeling moment, thriving and doing your very best to seize the moment and truly life, and enjoy the very best of yourself and your life.

SOS 27: The feel of a cigarette in your hand or mouth just feels so very uncomfortable and now for you, it's just plain wrong! You've moved on and are now and forever free and happy, moving forward in your life.

SOS 28: Completely relaxing into this and past and beyond any and all former barriers, you now and forever succeed and flow ever onward into a brighter and better life.

SOS 29: Each and every time you shake your head no, you are saying no to your past and moving into a better day. Each and every time you nod your head yes, you are saying yes to a newer and brighter, happier and better X *(smoke free, lighter, thinner, healthier and better you, etc)* chapter of your life. Now sure of yourself, you are unstoppable.

SOS 30: You are now smiling inside with a true and real knowing, glowing confidence. You are sure of yourself and certain of your improvements, more than any other time in your life.

SOS 31: Now that you know the truth, you are prevailing, dynamically and powerfully unstoppable in all that you seek to achieve. When you know the truth, you easily accomplish everything.

SOS 32: You are effectively finding ways of removing old past blockages, most especially relaxing deeper now and releasing the fear of [losing weight, change] and easily keeping it off, you are so mighty, powerful and effective at all of this, in fact it's easy.

SOS 33: Truly you have enjoyed this, your powerfully effective hypnosis session as only great, wonderful and beneficial improvements now come into your life from this, even in surprising and spectacularly beneficial ways just for you, powerfully improving all that you are, how you live and freeing up and powerfully activating only your very best effective inspirations and energies!

SOS 34: As everyone knows, once you have entered a brand new and better chapter of your life, things improve quickly and for only the very best. All things improve easily. You are so sure of yourself, that's where you are now and happily remain forever, in ever growing and glowing confidence. You are breaking through. You know you are truly unstoppable.

SOS 35: You might have once thought things impossible to improve or change, but you now think to yourself and know, "I now know I'm doing better and better and it's easy and amazingly simple." As always. my life is only getting better and better, I deserve this, it's now and forever mine and so it is.

SOS 36: You succeed easily, now finding even better motivated thoughts feelings and ideas, even finding excuses to succeed.

SOS 37: It's really just amazing how easy it is for you to just . . . (*melt off and keep off, 11, 26 and even 48 lbs. – remaining forever, smoke free, cigarette free, etc*).

SOS 38: You know, it's just amazing to realize right now, that you've relaxed your way into a newer and brighter better way, as the weight just seems to melt off and you easily lose now, XX pounds.

SOS 39: You are forever free of going to self-abusive extremes. Your new extreme, is to extremely take the very best care of yourself and to simply thrive, work out, sticking now in your favor to what you know works and just doing it, in amazing and even surprisingly easy ways.

SOS 40: You are now and forever forgiving and releasing all of the negative effects from your childhood, feeling upbeat even reinvented, having entered a brand new chapter of your life, so super motivated, all of your very best thoughts, feelings and supportive inspirations just rise to the top as the unwanted weight just seems to melt off you as you make the time to feel better about yourself and be motivated to break though and succeed easily and amazingly at this as never before.

SOS 41: All of the things in your life that ever once stood in your way have *Right Now*, just melted away and are gone. You are now and forever free to move on, excel and succeed at any and all things needed to improve your life.

SOS 42: The more in the past you once resisted yourself, the more in the future you work effectively in your favor to cleverly, abundantly and forever succeed at this. Nod your head yes for me because you know it's true.

SOS 43: In this brand new and better chapter of your life, you only thrive and succeed at this. You breakthrough easily and skillfully and even surprisingly – clever, fluid and adaptive success is your only option here, and you know that deeply and truly.

SOS 44: On each and every breath you take, and on each and every beat of your heart, you are released from past blockages that once ever stood in your way.

SOS 45: You are forgiven, now knowing you are feeling whole, happier and better. You are healing, you are healed, you are moving on in the very best and most supportive of ways.

SOS 46: Each and every thought, feeling, action or reaction is now working in your favor to improve your life.

SOS 47: You're smiling powerfully inside, with a warm knowing, glowing confidence. You can feel and now truly know that all old blockages and hindrances to your success are now just seemingly dissolving and melting away, as you have now moved into a new breakthrough chapter of your life. Feel that smile, nod your head yes. You really know you've succeeded here, out of your own way, you've succeeded, you are unstoppable, you are unbeatable, you are free, feeling fine!

SOS 48: With Cigarettes, you're just done and finished. You've moved on and into a forever healthier and better chapter of your life.

SOS 49: Right now you are free of any and all things toxic in your life, thoughts, feelings, memories, thought patterns, fears, worries and doubts. Now more correctly, more fluidly and powerfully unstoppable than ever before, you are thinking correctly and supportively, nurturingly and taking only the very best care of yourself, as your thoughts are now supporting you. Your feelings are pleasant and conducive to a happy life; happy memories are now supporting you.

SOS 50: You are feeling fine, wonderful, even fantastic. As if you've just had a 5 hour nap and 3 solid hours of full body massage. You are feeling fine, your body, emotions, thoughts and memories and feelings, even your spirit, in a new and more powerfully profound and optimized, fully functioning harmony, feeling truly and deeply better than wonderful and excellent, on top of your World.

Now and forever you are moving into the very best chapter of your life. Rising to the very top, you are thriving and succeeding, forever free of procrastination, activating and living your dreams and making them happen.

SOS 51: All things once toxic, are now released and resolved. All things once a hindrance, now are resolved and in their place. You are loved and supported, breaking through, freed, released and really wonderful as never before.

SOS 52: All things that once stressed you out or upset you are now easily handled and even vanquished by you.

SOS 53: Relax now barrier free and liberate new inspirations, allowing brighter, better and even brilliant ways of thinking acting, being and feeling to become a part of who you are. Melt and flow, relax and heal, get now inspired and allow a brilliant, new and more powerfully real series of new life supporting thoughts, feelings, habits, strategies and responses to forever emerge from your mind and into all that is your life. A brand new and better chapter of your life begins right now!

SOS 54: In fact, you might just come to now and forever know . . .

SOS 55: You know, it's almost funny. You are now and forever so very free now and free from smoking and cigarettes, so firmly entrenched in a happy, healthy and better life, smoke free, cigarette free, it seems like the previous chapter of your life was yesterday and yesterday really just seems now like a million years ago – it feels great to be so free, happy, healthy, content and safe, smoke free, cigarette free. You smile inside and you just know you are contented, serene, happy, very sure and safe.

SOS 56: Your new life now unfolds, in perfect and precise harmony, as you breakthrough here . . .

SOS 57: All things and energies that have ever worked against you are now and forever turned back upon themselves, to reduce, remove and completely eliminate those negative and destructive energies and their limitations, removing and eliminating difficulties, while ushering in a brand new and better chapter of your life, possibilities for victories, triumphs, and advances expand as you make and take bold strides, opening up your heart and your mind while magnetizing and liberating only the very best of experiences, breakthroughs, successes and events into your life.

SOS 58: Your powerful and adaptive mind is now creating flexible, clever, powerful and even surprisingly effective ways to dynamically and easily succeed at this. All of this, just getting easier and easier and more adaptive and more powerfully effective for you. You achieve and seize desired results with grace, ease and highest impact.

SOS 59: It has been said, that little steps mean a lot, this time you are assuredly easily succeeding at . . .

SOS 60: It's almost as if someone from deep inside of you in this moment, has reset a switch, the dial, a thermostat, or a computer of some type, easily allowing you to . . .

SOS 61: It's almost like someone from deep, deep inside of you in this moment, has opened a valve from deep, deep inside of you, draining away affectively any and all blockage and negativity energy, in fact, any and all shutouts are now easily been drained away.

What fills up the space right now, is a beautiful energy, and energy of inspired and creative life force, strength, adaptability, unconditional love, and inner light, which easily refills, in endless supply, focusing you, rejuvenating you, and liberating your unbeatable mighty inner hero.

SOS 62: Your mighty inner hero, a part of you that knows only strength, beyond doubt, remains fearless, courageous and mighty has now and forever effectively been activated from deep, deep inside of you right now, powerfully and effectively, creatively and dynamically, most adaptively and is right now working in your favor to achieve your well deserved and your very own ultimate success.

The part of you that is fully capable of saving children from great danger, like a fire or any other life threatening moments, is now actively working creatively and adaptively in your favor from deep, deep inside of you, to break you through right here and right now into a brand new, freer and better chapter of your life.

All of the negative, habitual, stagnating and limiting energies that once ever blocked you in any way, or ever once stood in your way are now cleverly and affectively turned back upon themselves as you adaptively and heroically breakthrough here with ultimate unbeatable success .

SOS 63: It's amazing to notice, how easy it is for you to win by releasing and resolving from your body, 9, 14, 23, 26, even 31 pounds.

SOS 64: You are taking any and all of this in stride, as a competent and skilled master of improvement of your life, easily and adaptively forever creating success within your life, for the greater the challenge the more liberated, safe, strong and mightier you become.

SOS 65: Each and every time you see a wrist watch, it seems to jump into your face, into your eyes, pleasantly surprising you, perhaps making you smile, giggle, or maybe even laugh, laugh out loud, just like a little kid, 8 years old, laughing at the funniest movie you ever saw, getting funnier and funnier.

Each and every time you look at your own wristwatch, you're more calm, and serene, more happy abundantly all over, more relaxed, and more assured of the very best chapter of your life beginning, one in which you are and you effectively remain, (smoke-free, cigarette-free – or – lighter, thinner, healthier, better, with a much higher metabolism, etc.).

[When the client laughs after being brought out of hypnosis at your wristwatch, they know something is taken place, something is different, and just maybe, important and forever life-changing improvements have taken place].

223

SOS 66: You smile to yourself and glow from places deep inside, knowing the truth of the new day, a new night and a better life.

SOS 67: You know it feels so great, to be feeling so truly wonderful, so vital, so complete, so alive, so completely alive, so sure of your life improvement, right here and right now, within such a pivotal place of power. So great to be alive, so full of life, and so full of vitality, while you are awake, while you are asleep, even while you were waking up, or even falling asleep.

SOS 68: For the mightier the challenge you ever once had, in a previous chapter of your life, now done, ever was, in this new chapter of your life, the more formidable and mighty you are and the more empty and nothing that former challenge now is, as you self-assuredly stand there proudly and laugh at how easy things have become.

SOS 69: You might even be feeling truly a thousand percent better, certain and sure, you have dynamically succeeded here in the most effective, dramatic and unstoppable of ways.

SOS 70: You quit smoking right now as if your life depended on it. Free and clear, happy and content, you've never felt so good!

SOS 71: Your mind now easily and powerfully generates any and all powerfully effective sensation or feeling, pace or plan, you now or will ever need to create adaptive and breakthrough success, in ways both known or unknown to you.

SOS 72: All former limitations, now resolved, you now and forever, unlimited.

SOS 73: You are certain and sure you are succeeding here unbeatably, even if only in your imagination, and as everyone knows, your imagination is here and now making it real.

SOS 74: You feel a release, you are released; forever freed, you right now know this to be true.

SOS 75: All of you now knowing a higher truth, as anything you put your mind to, now more easily than ever before within your grasp. Heroically freed, you now venture ever onward to seize your success and make it one with you, making success yours, while enjoying feelings of satisfaction and success, as a deep and true part of you now knows this and makes this all your very own. Having done all of the necessary work, succeeding brilliantly. The truth real, this is yours, certain and sure.

SOS 76: Your always clever and dynamic adaptive mind, is now working out beneficial ideas, methods, pathways, solutions, adaptations and improvements, to generate success in these ways. Most effectively and easily, generating complete and ultimate success, in ways both known and unknown to you, and so it is, and so it remains, and therefore you succeed.

SOS 77: You have already quit smoking as if your life depended on it, because it does, and so now you have, and you successfully remain, both now and forever, extending your life, and feeling wonderful.

SOS 78: Seizing the unstoppable inspiration in this moment and empowering yourself, you release barriers from the past and flow ever onward, ever more certain and self-assured knowing all of this to be true.

SOS 79: For in this new chapter of your life, the more mighty the challenge, the more determined you are to achieve your goals unbeatably, and so it remains in forever is.

SOS 80: You have set your mind to this, and you are doing better and better. For the greater challenge and circumstance, the mightier and more determined, the more heroically inspired you are, to breakthrough here unbeatably.

SOS 81: Your very best coming up to the surface now, all within your grasp, all within your ability and power to break you through here always and forever, and so it is and remains.

SOS 82: Your entire being now reset, re-tuned, recalibrated, in fact all of you is now and forever restoring, getting greater and greater physical shape. This newer, brighter, better, more empowered and inspired of your life.

You are now readily enjoying confidence and stamina to take any and all business to the next level, figuring out and activating new and limitlessly abundant levels of serenity and inner peace.

SOS 83: Taking better care of yourself, all things that once stood and your way, are and remain no longer.

SOS 84: All things once you're weakness, now your greatest strength.

SOS 85: Almost as if you've grown up just a little bit more, things of the past now done and finished, you now better and better feeling fine, empowered, inspired, unstoppable, goals achieved.

SOS 86: You have forever entered brand new chapter of your life. All of the adjustments necessary, all of the tweaks, any and all things necessary, have been reset, re-tuned, redefined, and improved in your favor, as you now and forever know this to be true but because and even in fact it is true from the deepest recesses inside of you.

Each and every aspect and area of your life, now working in a greater higher harmony, as the heroic and mighty inner master of your life that you are, from deepest places inside, is now automatically allowing this to happen, skillfully adjusting and adapting, only your very best, ways that serve you best and for those that you love the most, most especially yourself.

SOS 87:   Your automatic mind is now unstoppably making up its mind truly and forever remain just that way, smoke free, cigarette free, in the morning and throughout the rest of the day into the night, each and every day, each and every night.

SOS 88:   From deep, deep inside, you truly know, yesterday has taken care of you, and tomorrow will do just the same. All of your yesterdays have allowed you to learn or succeed, failure-free, and all of your tomorrows will be just the same.

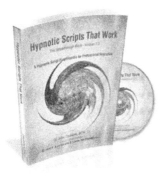
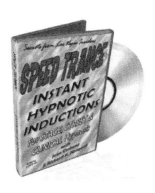
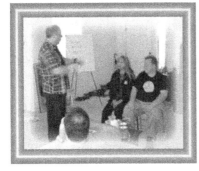

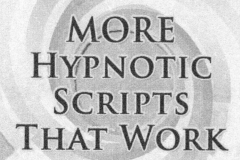
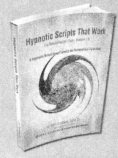

CPSIA information can be obtained
at www.ICGtesting.com
Printed in the USA
BVOW08s1702140318
510569BV00017B/894/P